Praise for
THE MIRACLE OF STEVIA

vides a wealth of research and information about the
, healthiest sweetener—and reveals the truth about as-
of the most dangerous. He also details the biased op-
he FDA to this herb and the illegal tactics the agency
ing to get it off the market. A commendable effort that
harassment going on in the nutritional supplement in-
y."

—Julian Whitaker, M.D., author of *Reversing Diabetes* and
publisher of *Health & Healing Newsletter*

"Stevias well-documented benefits as a noncaloric sweetener and
its virtual suppression make a great story, and probably no one
knows more about the properties and the politics of this remarkable herb than Jim May. The most comprehensive consumer book
on stevia ever published."

—Mark Blumenthal, founder and executive director of the
American Botanical Council and editor of *HerbalGram*

"*[The Miracle of Stevia]* tells it all. Perhaps most importantly, it pas-
sionately scrutinizes every piece of pertinent research on stevia and
brings into stark contrast the substantial documentation of the
safety of stevia against the pitiful attempts of big government and
industry to discredit the plant and paint it with an aura of potential
toxicity. Thanks to Jim, stevia is, and shall remain, one of the most
health-promoting materials in American homes."

—Daniel B. Mowrey, Ph.D., author of *Herbal Tonic Therapies,*
The Herbal Desk Reference, and
The Scientific Validation of Herbal Medicine

"Physicians and other healthcare professionals who deal with patients having diabetes, hypoglycemia, obesity, and heart disease are
constantly asked about 'sweet options' other than sugar, aspartame,
and saccharin. There is much to commend the use of stevia, which

to the best of my knowledge is both safe and probably beneficial. It is in this context that *The Miracle of Stevia* by James A. May is a unique amalgamation of extensive research, personal experiences, and constructive entrepreneurism that fills the existing void for an authoritative text on the subject."

—H. J. Roberts, M.D., F.A.C.P., F.C.C.P., author of
Aspartame Disease: An Ignored Epidemic and
Aspartame (NutraSweet): Is It Safe?

THE MIRACLE OF
STEVIA

Discover the Healing Power of Nature's Herbal Sweetener

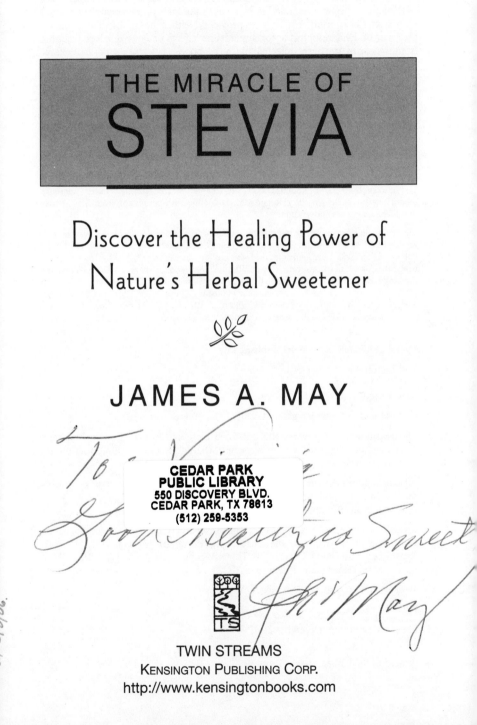

JAMES A. MAY

TWIN STREAMS
KENSINGTON PUBLISHING CORP.
http://www.kensingtonbooks.com

This book presents information based upon the research and personal experiences of the author. It is not intended to be a substitute for a professional consultation with a physician or other healthcare provider. Neither the publisher nor the author can be held responsible for any adverse effects or consequences resulting from the use of any of the information in this book. They also cannot be held responsible for any errors or omissions in the book. If you have a condition that requires medical advice, the publisher and author urge you to consult a competent healthcare professional.

Trademarked and registered names are used in an editorial fashion only in this book. Rather than put a trademark or registration symbol after every occurrence of such a name, we have printed the names with initial caps. These names are used in this book for the benefit of the trademark or registration owner and with no intention of infringement of the trademark or registration.

The quotes from H. J. Roberts, M.D., in Chapter 9 are reprinted from *Aspartame (NutraSweet): Is It Safe?* by H. J. Roberts, M.D. © 1990 with permission from The Charles Press, Philadelphia, Pennsylvania.

The recipes in Chapter 14 are reprinted from *Baking with Stevia: Recipes for the Sweet Leaf* by Rita DePuydt © 1997 with permission from Sun Coast Enterprises, Oak View, California; *Baking with Stevia II: More Recipes for the Sweet Leaf* by Rita DePuydt © 1998 with permission from Sun Coast Enterprises, Oak View, California; *The Stevia Cookbook: Cooking with Nature's Calorie-Free Sweetener* by Ray Sahelian, M.D., and Donna Gates © 1999 with permission from Avery, a division of Penguin-Putnam Publishing Group, New York; and *Stevia Sweet Recipes: Sugar-Free—Naturally!* (Second Edition) © 1999 by Jeffrey Goettemoeller with permission from Vital Health Publishing, Ridgefield, Connecticut.

TWIN STREAMS BOOKS are published by

Kensington Publishing Corp.
850 Third Avenue
New York, NY 10022

All Kensington titles, imprints and distributed lines are available at special quantity discounts for bulk purchases for sales promotion, premiums, fund-raising, educational or institutional use.

Special book exceprts or customized printings can also be created to fit specific needs. For details, write or phone the office of the Kensington Special Sales Manager: Kensington Publishing Corp., 850 Third Avenue, New York, NY 10022. Attn. Special Sales Department. Phone: 1-800-221-2647.

Twin Streams and the TS logo Reg. U.S. Pat. & TM Off.

ISBN 0-7582-0220-2

First Trade Printing: December 2003
10 9 8 7 6 5 4 3 2

Printed in the United States of America

This book is affectionately dedicated to my wife, Carol, and to my sons and daughters, who were deprived of much that should have been theirs as I struggled against nearly insurmountable odds to learn about stevia and the other healing herbs of Paraguay, and to bring them to the United States.

Carol watched in desperation as our financial resources dwindled. "Dad" was not able to be in attendance at many of the important activities of the children as they grew up. They could not understand why they could not have all of the "nice things" that their friends enjoyed.

My children are now adults and, I believe, will all agree that if this book helps you to receive the blessings of improved health and well-being that can come from stevia, their sacrifice will have been worth the cost.

CONTENTS

FOREWORD

My father, Arthur, is a type 2 diabetic. My uncles Joey and Eddie were diabetics and my cousin Alan, who is my age, has been on insulin for more than two decades. My paternal grandmother, Anna, for whom I am named, died from diabetic complications at the age of thirty-nine.

Do I take diabetes personally? Oh, yes. You bet I do.

And so when Jim May asked me to write the foreword for his book, *The Miracle of Stevia*, I was very pleased. Not only does stevia provide extraordinary healing benefits for a number of seemingly unrelated conditions and ailments (hypertension, low immunity, fatigue, burns, cuts, skin conditions, and bleeding gums) but the latest research suggests that it is so instrumental in normalizing blood sugar levels that it may soon be used for diabetics as a medication. Now, that alone speaks volumes about the power of this tiny green plant originally from the rain forests of Paraguay and Brazil whose leaves are 200 to 400 times sweeter than sugar.

Stevia is now also grown in Korea, Thailand, China, and Japan, where it has been put to exceptionally good use as a sweetener in beverages and foods. In fact, stevia makes up almost 50 percent of the sweetener market in Japan these days, where it is used in "diet" drinks rather than the artificial sweeteners that permeate America's soft drinks, beverages, and instant iced teas.

But amazing healing and sweetening benefits aside, let's talk about taste for a moment. While researching the various natural sweeteners on the market for my book *The Fat Flush Plan*, I taste-tested many different brands of stevia, only to find that while they may indeed be healthful for the body, their aftertaste is so unpleasant that I questioned who would really use them on a regular basis. Besides, the unusual aftertaste I found with various stevia products on the market today just doesn't lend itself to my Fat Flush smoothies and desserts.

I finally settled on SteviaPlus (the "Plus" being inulin or fructooligosachharides from chicory roots, which are nourishing to the friendly flora in the gastrointestinal tract) because it simply tastes so much better than any other brand I tried with my taste-testing focus groups. But the most important test of all came when I gave the little green packets to my father who, when he put a dash into his herbal tea, for the first time didn't make the face as he usually does with anything natural.

Probably just as meaningful to me as the benefits of SteviaPlus are the achievements and vision of its creator, Jim May. I never met this fine gentleman before I wrote about his product in my book. I have since, however, gotten to know him and am very impressed and inspired by his vision for stevia—from wanting to wipe out diabetes among the Native American tribes to reducing world hunger in underdeveloped nations.

Within the pages of this book, *The Miracle of Stevia,* you will learn much about this brave and valiant man who fought the Food and Drug Administration and won in making stevia available as a dietary or nutritional supplement so that we all could enjoy its healing benefits here in the United States.

I know you will enjoy this book, become fascinated (as I did) with Jim May's personal story, and look forward to experimenting with stevia, too.

—Ann Louise Gittleman, Ph.D.
Author of the *New York Times* bestseller *The Fat Flush Plan*

INTRODUCTION

For years, stevia advocates have encouraged me to write a book about the healing benefits of this and other herbs of South America. I was afraid to do so. In the United States of America—the land of the free—the Food and Drug Administration (FDA) does not allow anyone who sells a food or herb to make statements about its healing benefits or positive effects against diseases. You cannot write about them. You cannot speak about them to a group or to an individual. To do so and then offer to sell the herb or food by its brand name can lead to possible confiscation of product, computers, and assets, and even arrest and imprisonment. You will be accused of practicing medicine without a license or selling un-approved drugs.

These rules and regulations, strictly enforced by the FDA, are based upon a law passed by Congress in 1938, which was back in the days of ignorance regarding the nutritional benefits of food and the functioning of the human body. That section of the Federal Food, Drug and Cosmetic Act states that any substance or "article intended to diagnose, treat, mitigate, cure or prevent disease in man or animal" is a drug and is therefore under the strict control of the FDA. In 1938 this statement was merely a reflection of the ignorance of the times. Today, I believe it is an inexcusable crime against the health and well-being of all mankind.

We now possess much more knowledge about the human body and the interrelationship and interdependence of its glands, organs, tissues, nervous system, and even cells, which in and of themselves possess an intelligence. The human body is an incredible electrical, electromagnetic, hydroelectrical, chemical, self-lubricating, self-regulating, and self-regenerating masterpiece. Its component parts are totally interrelated and self-communicating. It is fueled, repaired, and maintained by a combination of the nutrients assimilated from the foods we eat, the water we drink, the air we breathe, and the thoughts we think. Scientists are learning about the wondrous effects of the vitamins, minerals, and vast array of phytochemicals contained within plants and herbs upon the structure, function, health, and well-being of the body. We now know that certain nutrients, controlled thought impulses, and even the state of mind stimulate improved activity of the immune system. Other nutrients nourish various glands, organs, and friendly organisms dwelling within us, thereby improving their function and viability. This adjusts the volume of vital chemicals and specific nutrients these glands produce, as required to maintain or improve the health and vitality of the whole body. To deny access to truthful information about the healing benefits of fluids, foods, herbs, and mental activity, whether it is modern science or ancient folklore, is a terrible injustice against the citizens of America, Europe, and the world.

WHERE IS TRUTH? WHERE IS WISDOM?

Before my own personal experiences with the healing herbs of Paraguay, I worked in the medical field and believed that the use of herbs was quackery. I had spent fifteen years developing the artificial organ and kidney transplant programs in Arizona, and serving as a consultant throughout the United States to hospitals, physicians, and the manufacturers of dialysis equipment and supplies. I was a consultant to the chief of the End Stage Renal Disease Bureau, in Baltimore, Maryland, which was the federal government's regulating body for this medical therapy. Through private medical care corporations, to which I was a consultant or which I helped organize and develop, I was involved in new innovations and methodologies in patient care and the invention of better equipment, machines, and facilities to perform dialysis. With this background I was convinced that the only routes to healing were through medical intervention, including pharmaceuticals, coupled with faith. I was wrong.

I have always possessed a deep and abiding faith in God as a loving, caring Heavenly Father, who is concerned about the physical and spiritual welfare of His children during our mortal sojourn upon this planet called Earth. These past twenty years have enabled me to understand that our Creator has also placed upon Earth, primarily in the plant world, the cure for all diseases and illnesses that beset mankind through natural causes. It has become clear to me that our first four lines of defense against disease and illness should be:

1. Exercising wisdom in what we take into our bodies. We must understand that every substance that enters our body, regardless of whether it is through our mouth, nose, skin, eyes, ears, or mind, produces a lasting effect upon us, for good or ill, for health or sickness.

2. Eating, and enjoying the aroma and the taste of wholesome and nutritious foods, including herbs, as close to their natural forms as possible, for the nourishment and strengthening of the body and the prevention of disease.

3. Assisting our body in mobilizing the warriors of our immune system when viruses or harmful bacteria invade our body, or when we just think we have been exposed to them, and sending them forth into battle more rapidly and better armed, by ingesting certain foods and herbs.

4. Exercising the positive and powerful mental action called faith. In and of itself, faith has an incredible effect upon the body and its internal workings. Simply stated, faith is the ability to use our minds to effect change within ourselves and the physical

world of which we are a part and which surrounds us, whether people or things. It is the moving cause, or principle underlying all action. It is the prerequisite for the ability to perform a task, the power to achieve.

To discount the power of the human mind upon the functions of the body is foolishness. The human body was designed to respond automatically to sight, aroma, taste, nutrients in foods, and mental thoughts. You are what you smell, breathe, drink, eat, absorb through your skin, hear, see, feel with your emotions, and think. Persons who deny that each one of these pathways into the body profoundly affects the body and the brain for good or ill languish in the realms of foolishness and self-deceit.

THE MEDICAL EYE BEGINS TO OPEN AFTER ITS LONG SLUMBER

Although many scientists refuse to admit it, much of what is considered scientific fact or truth in reality is nothing more than the folklore of scientists and medical doctors. They are adamant about what they "know" but they are wrong. They often misinterpret and therefore misunderstand new "discoveries" and their effects on the human body. When the truth is discovered, they often reject it until some brave soul comes along who possesses the courage to do battle with the scientific establishment and its "known facts." Arrogant ignorance often requires many years, even decades, and sometimes generations to become enlightened with truth. The paradigm of thought of the "expert" is often his or her greatest weakness. However, with one eye struggling to open and beginning to see, even if only dimly, through the cloudy matter of medical superstition, perhaps in time both eyes will open wide and, with clear vision, behold reality.

Millions of people suffer mild to severe health problems because of ignorance. They simply do not know that there are natural foods, herbs, and nutritional supplements that would bring them great relief and often healing, *with no harmful side effects.* Man-made drugs are not always necessary. They may not even be the best method of safe therapy. The bureaucracies of government often deny consumers access to vital information that could significantly improve their health and benefit their lives. Sometimes this is out of ignorance but often, I suspect, it is done to protect the pharmaceutical and medical industries, which spend enormous amounts of money on lobbying and advertising efforts to protect and expand their highly profitable positions in the arena of disease management.

For many decades medical doctors vehemently denied the need for anyone to supplement his or her diet with vitamins and minerals. To add vitamins and minerals to one's normal diet, they said, was unnecessary. However, on April 6, 1992, *Time* magazine valiantly took on the medical establishment with a bold cover story titled "The New Scoop on Vitamins." The teaser declared, "They may be much more important than doctors thought in warding off cancer, heart disease and the ravages of aging—and, no, you may not be getting enough of these crucial nutrients in your diet."

However, as the article suggested, the medical establishment was not yet ready to accept what was becoming incredibly obvious to everyone else:

> But for every true believer in the power of vitamins . . . there is an agnostic, a skeptic who insists that vitamins are the opiate of the people. Among the doubters are many doctors. They have been persuaded by decades of public health pronouncements, endorsed by the U.S. National Academy of Sciences and the National Institutes of Health, that claim people can get every nutrient they need from the food they eat. Popping vitamins "doesn't do you any good," sniffs Dr. Victor Herbert, a professor of medicine at New York City's Mount Sinai medical school. "We get all the vitamins we need in our diets. Taking supplements just gives you expensive urine."[1]

However, in the year 2002 the doctors who control the American Medical Association (AMA) changed their opinion on the need for supplementation and now suggest that everyone take vitamins daily to prevent disease and improve their health and vitality. In a research review published in the June 19, 2002 issue of the prestigious

Journal of the American Medical Association (JAMA), two Harvard researchers reported finding a direct association between inadequate intakes of certain vitamins and the increased risk for chronic conditions such as coronary heart disease, cancer, and osteoporosis. They had searched a database of 11 million indexed journal citations published over a period of thirty-six years.[2] The June 26, 2002, issue included two studies that indicated that antioxidant intake may reduce the risk of Alzheimer's disease by up to 70 percent.[3] Studies continue to mount linking nutritional supplements to disease prevention, and are flooding the pages of scientific journals (see Chapter 6). Perhaps someday doctors will also come to understand that many of the drugs that the manufacturers entice them to prescribe are not only unnecessary but more harmful to the human body than the condition or disease for which they are administered.

In twenty-five years or so, our children and grandchildren will look back upon the late 1900s with well-deserved disdain, disgust, and perhaps abhorrence. They will correctly declare that notwithstanding our wonderful advances in science, our civilization was both ignorant and barbaric owing to the way disease was treated, mistreated, and possibly even invented by the drug companies to increase the sale of prescription drugs. Hopefully, they will fondly remember the first decade of the 2000s as the beginning of the Age of Medical Enlightenment, at least when it comes to the human body and its requirement for quality nutrition to both prevent and heal disease and to achieve vibrant health and well-being. With all of this new knowledge being distilled upon us, like the biblical manna from Heaven, we must ask: Has the FDA neither eyes to see, nor ears to hear? The 1938 law, based on ignorance and promulgated in greed, must be changed. It must be tempered with the knowledge that exists today concerning how mental activity, emotions, water, vitamins, minerals, enzymes, and other macronutrients and micronutrients contained in various foods, especially raw, unprocessed foods, and whole herbs affect the health and vitality of the human body. Foods and the nutrients they contain are not drugs. They are the fuels of health, the essentials of life.

WHY YOU NEED THIS BOOK

As you read *The Miracle of Stevia,* you will understand why the events I relate herein need to be told. Without understanding that they really did occur, it might be hard for you to believe the vendetta that I believe a major U.S. corporation in the artificial sweetener industry and the FDA have waged against the totally innocent stevia. As you proceed, you will come to understand the poem "Stevia's Lament" on pages 12–13.

The Roman author Terentianus Maurus, who lived around A.D. 200, wrote this insightful statement: "Books have their own destiny." The purpose of this book is to inform you about stevia, its uses, and its benefits to the health and well-being of the human organism. *You have the right to know.*

My information comes from four sources:

1. Personal experience, owing to the healing that members of my family and I have directly experienced.

2. The Guarani people of Paraguay, who have used stevia daily for more than 1,500 years.

3. The thousands of people, including physicians and nutritionists, who have called, written, or come to see me, from the length and breadth of America, just to relate their own healing experience with stevia and/or other Paraguayan herbs. (I will not use the real names of these people. Experience has demonstrated that other people, upon learning their names and seeking validation for their own trial of the herbs, inundate them with telephone calls.)

4. The published scientific research papers, which I have studied.

After writing this list, I became fascinated that I had four sources of learning about stevia. To the ancient Hebrew Prophets of the Old Testament, and also to John, as he outlined in his prophetic book, the Revelation, four was a symbolic number relating to aspects of wholeness or completeness. Such is the destiny of stevia. You will understand my intrigue with this as we continue together on this fascinating journey of learning and potential healing. I trust our voyage will be as enjoyable as it is informative.

ANECDOTAL EVIDENCE VERSUS SCIENCE

Those people whose business is the manufacture, marketing, or prescribing of drugs and medical intervention loudly proclaim that valid information on the efficacy of a drug comes only from medical research and double-blind studies. They deny the value of the actual experiences of living human beings—no matter how many people have benefited, or how long the substance has been in effective use by various cultures. They term such real-life experiences "only anecdotal." What this really means is that even though the food, herb, medicine, or supplement may be effective with people, its effectiveness has not been "proven" by scientists, inuring to their personal fame and to the profit of the medical and pharmaceutical industries. Because they do not understand how it works or why it is effective, it does not exist. However, truth is truth, regardless of its source!

For the past thirty-five years I have served my fellow man in the fields of both medicine and herbs. I have personally witnessed the harm—and deaths—caused by the side effects of FDA-approved drugs, prescribed and administered by medical doctors. I have also had thousands of people relate to me their own personal stories of healing with natural herbs. I have concluded that I prefer the anecdotal "wisdom of the ancients." The ancients relied upon the healing and health-promoting compounds found naturally, in their proper balance, in the leaves, roots, bark, and flowers of various plants. But because I also sell the herbs, I was forbidden to tell or publish what I have learned. It does not matter that millions of South Americans and tens of thousands of North Americans claim to have experienced the healing benefits. Fortunately times are changing. A better-informed public is now demanding the inalienable right to know more.

In stark contrast, medical authorities hide from the public the fact that recent studies have estimated that more than 100,000 people die annually in hospitals in the United States as a direct result of the FDA-approved drugs given them, as prescribed by their physicians, and used as directed. Further, these deaths are unrelated to the original illness. Almost daily we read or hear reports of terrible, life-threatening side effects of FDA-approved drugs that are touted on television and on the written page directly to the consuming public, as if they were an "elixir of life." Without their drugs, the commercials imply, you cannot enjoy life, nor find love or happiness. These 100,000 deaths (that are reported) make the 107 deaths caused by Elixir of Sulfanilamide in 1937, which you will learn about in Chapter 12, pale into virtual insignificance. When you have finished reading Chapter 12, you might ask yourself, "Where are the FDA heroes of today?"

WHY STEVIA IS NOT SOLD AS A FOOD OR SWEETENER

Petitions to have stevia approved as a food or sweetener, or added to the FDA's Generally Recognized as Safe (GRAS) list, have been submitted several times by various individuals and organizations. Two of these petitions were introduced by large credible organizations. One was submitted by the Lipton Tea Company, which wanted to use the leaves to sweeten its teas, thus requiring no sugar or artificial sweeteners to be added to the finished beverage by the consumer. The second petition was submitted by the American Herbal Products Association (AHPA), on behalf of its member companies. Approval would have allowed manufacturers to use stevia both to sweeten and to enhance the flavor of their finished products. This would have provided consumers with much better tasting "health foods." The FDA refused to "file" the petitions. To do so would have required public comment, which would have necessitated that the public be informed about stevia. An attempt was also made to have stevia "grandfathered" in as GRAS, under a ruling that substances in common use prior to 1958 could not be disallowed. The FDA's position was that stevia was not known or in use prior to 1958, except by a very small group of Guarani Indians living in the rain forests of Paraguay, and thus it did not qualify under the grandfather clause.

The FDA also states that stevia may not be safe for human consumption if used as a sweetener or food product. This book will enable you to thoroughly examine the scientific validity of these safety issues. You will see that the FDA's safety concern is totally unexplainable and inexplicable when compared with the ruling it made regarding the redefinition and approval of the substance called aspartame (NutraSweet, Equal) for use as a sweetener. This was done by the FDA commissioner in direct opposition to the testimony of food scientists and medical doctors, and, in my opinion, in complete disregard for the harm and potential medical crises that would inevitably be inflicted upon a large number of unwary consumers. In Chapter 6, you will learn why this substance, masquerading as a sweetener, causes fat gain, not weight loss.

As you read this book, I invite you to be the jury regarding the FDA's position on these matters. The FDA was created to protect the public from harmful substances, specifically man-made drugs and nonfood fillers that are used in foods to enhance volume, not to interfere with natural foods that are not harmful, especially those that are beneficial to health and well-being. Perhaps you will agree that the FDA, as it functions today, fits the definition ascribed to a radical organization, which, I submit, is an organization that, having lost sight of the purpose of its existence, intensifies its efforts to the detriment of others, including those it was supposed to serve.

Perhaps, you will also come to the conclusion that an agency of the government that makes rules and regulations should never also have the authority to enforce them. I believe that this is the very power that breeds corruption and tyranny.

OPPORTUNITY CALLS

When the health editor of a New York City publishing firm called and indicated an interest in having me write a book about stevia, I was delighted! I realized that if this third party published the book, consumers could be truthfully informed about stevia, as long as the information was generic—that is, about the herb, and not about my specific brand of stevia products. Therefore, my intent in this book is to inform, to educate, and to enlighten you about both the healing benefits and the sweetening properties of stevia in its various generic forms, including when and how to use them. Be aware, however, that there are numerous forms of stevia available in the marketplace under various brand names. These products range from very poor to excellent. "Let the buyer beware" applies to stevia in all of its forms. All of my experiences with stevia involve the products produced by my own company. I cannot attest to the quality, and thus, the effectiveness of other brands of stevia. However, that is not meant to imply that other brands of stevia products may not be as effective as mine.

My twenty years of experience with stevia are unique. Owing to my experience, many people have suggested that I possess more actual knowledge about the healing benefits of the various forms of stevia than any other person living today. Since no one else in this industry has had similar experiences with stevia, perhaps they are correct. You be the judge. It is my firm belief that you, or someone in your family, can enjoy improved health and well-being from stevia, either by eating or drinking it, applying it to the skin, or both.

As you read about the "miracles" that are attributed to the use of one form or another of stevia, you may, at first, be inclined to doubt such possibilities. We have all been well indoctrinated by the pharmaceutical industry. However, there are scientific explanations for these "miracles." As you learn about the vast array of vitamins, minerals, and other phytonutrients that exist in stevia, in their appropriate and natural balance, and their effect upon both the cells and the tissues of the human body, you will begin to understand. Then when you see how stevia inhibits the growth of, and even destroys, many of the viruses and harmful bacteria that invade our bodies, it all will become wonderfully clear. Be patient, and let the knowledge of stevia's healing benefits gently distill upon you.

Stevia is extraordinarily sweet. Nearly all of the scientific research and individual experimentation with stevia have been to prove its safety as a sweetener. The healing benefits, although noted by the scientists, have been "sidebars." Major food and drug corporations, and thus the FDA, have been interested in stevia only as a sugar substitute. That, they believe, is where the big profits are. The objective of a least one corporation in the artificial sweetener industry has been to either take control of stevia or keep it out of the marketplace. It has not been aware of the ability of stevia to heal the body.

Thus we have the poem "Stevia's Lament," on pages 12–13, which encapsulates the story of stevia, my own experiences, and those of others, from 1982 until the present date.

John Naisbitt, author of the bestselling book *Megatrends 2000* (Avon, 1999), said, "Communications and information are entertainment, and if you don't understand that, you're not going to communicate." I shall try very hard to communicate by making this book both highly informative and very entertaining. I intend to tell my story and reveal myself to a degree not previously undertaken. While I will mention a few of the other healing herbs of the rain forests of Paraguay as they relate to stevia and to my introduction to it, this book is about *The Miracle of Stevia*.

 ## Stevia's Lament

> *Beast of favored secret lair*
> *With fierceness did arise,*
> *To observe the approach*
> *Of the innocent, the unwise.*
>
> *"Who doth disturb my serenity,*
> *The sweetness of my territory?*
> *Who seeks to glean a measure*
> *Of my fortune and my glory?"*
>
> *"I seek neither fortune nor fame,*
> *Only healing for son and daughter."*
> *Sneering lip, nostrils aflame, cowardly plan.*
> *"I'll roast him for my fodder."*
>
> *Beastly preserve, approached by others*
> *Eager to bask in terrain so sweet.*

Breath on fire, ghastly roar.
Trespassers in required retreat.

Likened not unto warriors brave,
In fables long since told.
These timid ones possess no shield,
No weapon to battle beast so bold.

With sword and shield, who will stand
And save my helpless little ones?
Who will slay the dragon fierce,
And rescue, fearful, frightened sons?

Who can withstand the powerful glare
Of beast and servant in union unholy?
Who will brave the breath of fire
And extinguish the servant's horrid folly?

"Here am I! Here are we!"
Shout journalist, doctor, politician.
Pen is mightier than sword,
"We accept the glorious mission."

1

An Unbeliever Learns About Herbs That Heal the Body

"To know what you know, and to know what you don't know,
is the characteristic of one who knows."
—Confucius (551–479 B.C.), Chinese philosopher

In 1966, I accepted a position at Good Samaritan Hospital in Phoenix, Arizona, as administrator of the newly developing End Stage Renal Disease Program and simultaneously with the Arizona Kidney Foundation as administrator of the organization. No one had the faintest idea of what my job at the hospital should entail. It had never before existed—anywhere in the United States. I was hired at the insistence of the doctors treating kidney disease and turned loose to discover on my own how to organize, develop, and manage a kidney dialysis/transplantation program, at that time considered experimental, and make it financially viable for the hospital. It was an awesome task, but I was supported by excellent physicians, registered nurses, and medical staff. In those early days, we were literally discovering the path and then uncovering it for others to follow.

By the late 1970s, I was considered the foremost expert in America in my now rapidly developing profession. I served as a consultant to physicians, hospitals, dialysis facilities, architects designing innovative treatment centers, corporations inventing and manufacturing medical equipment and supplies, and the chief of the End Stage Renal Disease Program of the federal government. I stood on what had become familiar and very solid ground.

VENTURE INTO THE UNKNOWN

In 1980, I joined a corporation that developed and managed dialysis centers on a national basis. By the time we opened the fourth dialysis center, the owners had received a lucrative offer from a national chain of for-profit hospitals. They sold. In 1982, I found it necessary to resign my position with the hospital organization following a dispute over billing practices being instituted that I considered unethical.

Not long thereafter, I was in my study reflecting on my recent action and my total loss of income, and the impact on my family, which consisted of my wife and five children, the oldest of whom was ready to enter high school. My wife had returned to college to obtain an advanced degree. My previous hospital position had long since been filled. What would I do now? Where could I find employment? During my mental deliberations the phone rang. It was a friend whom I had recently met, inviting me to his home. This friend, whom I'll call E. E., wanted me to meet "a very interesting young man" with whom he had become acquainted. With nothing better to do that evening, I accepted the invitation.

The visit was pleasant enough. The young man, whom I'll call H. H., had just arrived from Paraguay, where he had been serving in the Peace Corps. During the course of our conversation he began to make what I considered to be outrageous and ridiculous statements. He claimed that the Guarani Indians of Paraguay had herbs from which they made a tea that "would cure the flu in one day." With some degree of arrogance I told him, "That's absurd! Herbal remedies are nothing but quackery and the result of ignorance among uneducated people."

He persisted. I resisted. Finally, in some degree of desperation and indignation, he reached into his briefcase and pulled out a small cellophane bag of green leaves. He put one leaf in his mouth, as did my friend. He then offered one to me. Not knowing what it was and having become suspicious of his judgment, I said, "No thanks, I don't put strange leaves in my mouth."

Both he and my friend insisted that I taste one. Together, they finally overcame my objections, insisting that the leaf was neither a drug nor harmful. At length I put a leaf to my lips and gingerly tasted it. I then put it into my mouth and fully enjoyed the delicately sweet flavor. The longer I held it in my mouth, the sweeter it became. It was delicious! That was my introduction to premium-quality Paraguayan stevia leaves. Though I did not know it at that moment, my life and destiny were changed forever.

The delicious taste of stevia had cracked the doorway to my mind ever so slightly. H. H. then began to present me with Japanese research concerning stevia, its safety, and its extraordinarily sweet extract, called stevioside. Japanese interest in stevia had intensified by 1970 when the Japanese National Institute of Health had taken plants back to Japan and begun a scientific investigation. Japanese scientists had developed and patented extraction methods to remove the intensely sweet compounds from the leaves. While good-quality stevia leaves can be 30 times sweeter than sugar, their various sweet constituents, called glycosides, can be 250 to 400 times sweeter than sugar and contain *no calories*. By 1980, stevioside was in use as *the* sweetener, alone or blended with other sweeteners, in soft drinks, chewing gum, ice cream, orange juice, soy sauce, and hundreds of other food products throughout Japan. It had also been discovered that stevioside enhances the appearance of frozen foods. The researchers predicted that stevioside was destined to become the commercial sweetener of choice in Japan and eventually the world.

In 1982, when America was searching for a safe alternative to sugar and cyclamates, these statistics were impressive. I was hooked. I reasoned that with such a wonderfully sweet and healthful product, it would not be overly difficult to find an interested individual or corporation with the funds necessary to introduce stevia into the United States. Wrong again.

Before the evening was over, I had given E. E. and H. H. a check amounting to nearly all of my life's savings. The three of us would set up a business to manufacture and market stevia leaf products and stevia extracts. H. H. was to return to Paraguay, send us stevia leaves, and run the operation there. E. E. and I would locate the right partners and, with sufficient funding, develop manufacturing operations and market the products.

Can you imagine the reaction of my wife, the next morning,

when I told her that I had given our life savings to a young man whom I had just met, and who was now on his way to Paraguay? I'll never forget it! Without belaboring the painful details, I soon learned E. E. used some of my money for his personal benefit and was out looking for another small-time sucker to invest in stevia.

What had I gotten myself into? This, I realized, had been one of those experiences when deep inner feelings overcame the restraints and cautions of the mind. I decided that if I ever heard from H. H., and if he really intended to send me the stevia leaves, I would tell him to also send me the leaves he said would cure the flu. I did not believe it possible, but by this time I had determined that I had better salvage whatever I could. Perhaps my wife was right. We'd never see our money again.

As the days passed, my concern deepened. Had E. E. and H. H. deceived me somehow and the leaves really weren't that sweet? Had they dipped them in a honey solution? While I deliberated upon my situation, I put a few leaves in a glass of ice water, waited two or three minutes, and took a swallow. It wasn't sweet. My last vestige of hope plummeted. Now worry really set in. Then the phone rang. After about fifteen minutes of conversation, I was thirsty and reached for the glass of cool water. It was so sweet I nearly spewed it out on the carpet. It was incredible. I was so exhilarated I could hardly finish the conversation. Obviously, stevia leaves release their sweet glycosides quickly in hot water but very slowly in cold water.

As fortune would have it, H. H. did call a few days later and was delighted when I asked for the leaves that "cured" the flu. Within several weeks, however, I became concerned that H. H. also was not being honest with me, even as he complained that E. E. had deceived us both. I began to fear that he, too, was trying to slip me a lemon. If so, I was determined to somehow make lemonade. Well, at least I could add stevia to my lemonade and forget the sugar. But that's the rest of my story.

ANCIENT LEAVES THAT "CURE" THE FLU

Within a few weeks of my original meeting with E. E. and H. H., I received several large bags of leaves. Now what was I to do?

Unfortunately, or fortunately, I came down with a case of the flu. At that time my immune system was not functioning well. I had been on strong allergy medications, including cortisone injections, for more than thirty-five years and they had taken their toll. Without a well-functioning and rapidly responding immune system, when a flu virus attacked me, I got really sick. Episodes would last ten days or longer. I decided to try the leaves from Paraguay.

Having never made a cup of tea in my life, I was not sure what to do. But H. H. had said to put a handful of Amba-y leaves, a handful Yaguarundi leaves, and a handful of stevia leaves in two quarts of water and sip the resulting tea throughout the day until it was gone. I boiled the leaves for about ten minutes. The taste was not great and the smell was worse, but I was committed. I woke up the next morning completely well. I felt great! I could not believe it. This was impossible! It just couldn't happen. "Obviously," I thought to myself, "I didn't have the flu, because leaves can't do that." Some of us are really hardheaded—or brainwashed.

Reflecting back on those early days of my skepticism, I think that the Lord above decided to teach Jim May an important lesson. This mortal skeptic had to learn an important truth. About two weeks following this first experience with the leaves from Paraguay, I woke up with the severest episode of flu that I had ever experienced in my life. I had a high fever, a severely sore throat, and a painful earache. My eyes hurt. I was nauseous. I ached in every joint and muscle of my body. When I tried to sit up, I became dizzy. I was miserable. But I had so much to do. I had to find permanent employment. There was no time for a two-to-three-week illness.

Prayer had always been an important part of my life, and I prayed that God would bless me and heal me. He had done so before and I had faith He would help me now. Following my pattern, having asked for Divine assistance, I now needed to get to a doctor and receive an injection of penicillin and appropriate medications. "I'm too sick to waste time with those leaves," I reasoned. Then those never-to-be-forgotten words entered my mind: "You are to use the leaves from Paraguay."

"But I'm too sick for that," was my mental response.

"Use the leaves. Get up and make the beverage."

Previous experiences in my life had taught me to obey without question when the Divine impulses came into my mind. This time, I suppose, I was so ill that rational thought escaped me. I resisted, thinking that I was just too sick for experimentation. The voice within my mind continued to repeat the instructions. At length, I realized that if I was to have any mental peace, I must try the leaves for one day. Then I would go to the doctor.

My wife and children had gone to school. I struggled to get out of bed, but was so dizzy that I had to hold on to the dresser. Slowly, I made my way to the kitchen, balancing myself on furniture as I staggered along. I found a pot, added the leaves and two quarts of water, and put it on the stove to cook. After boiling the leaves, steeping them, and cooling the brew a little, I poured the tea through a strainer, dumped the leaves back into the water, and forced myself to drink a glassful of the warm liquid. (Later, during my first trip to Paraguay, I would learn how to sip this and other healing herbal teas through a *bombilla*, which strains out the leaf particles.) Then I reasoned, I'm so sick, maybe I should chew the leaves and get everything possible out of them. I fished some of the leaves out of the pot and chewed them until there was no flavor left, and then trashed the residue. I returned to bed and quickly fell into a deep sleep.

When I awakened about three hours later, I repeated the procedure. Again I fell into a deep sleep. I repeated this process throughout the day. I was preparing more tea when my wife, Carol, came home to check on me. "What have you done to my kitchen?" she asked. "It smells awful in here!" I didn't know it smelled. I couldn't smell. And besides, I was feeling better and didn't care if it smelled. That night, my sleep was deep and undisturbed.

When I awakened early the next morning, I was totally well. Not a single symptom of the flu remained. I could hardly believe it possible. This time, however, there was no question. I had had a very severe case of the flu. The leaves from Paraguay had worked! I was completely cured in just one day. I felt wonderful! The Guarani Indians had aptly named the herbal tea *O´ Ho´ Mguara!* This means "It must go!" They had named the beverage for the results it obtained. I wondered if the tea would work that well with others, or if it was just because I had followed the prompting that had come into my mind.

The next day I told a close friend about my experience. After all, it was just too incredible to keep to myself. Within a few days his wife called. He was sick with the flu. "Can we have some of those leaves that cured your flu?" Tess asked. "Byron is so sick, and if he doesn't go to work, he won't earn any commissions and we won't be able to make our house payment." She didn't really need to exert such pressure. I was anxious to see if he would have the same experience. By this time I had called H. H. in Paraguay and told him of my experience. When I related how bad the kitchen had smelled, he was incredulous. "Don't you know how to make tea?" No, I didn't. I had never drunk tea, let alone made it. He explained exactly how to prepare the beverage. The leaves should never be boiled, just steeped for about ten minutes in water that is hot enough to give off steam. The next time I made O´ Ho´ Mguara, I followed his instructions. The beverage produced no bad smell, just a very slight, but pleasant aroma of licorice.

Having learned the correct method of preparation, I took some leaves to my friends and explained to Tess how to make the tea. Byron was well and at work the next day. But now Tess had the flu. She made more tea, drank it, and was well in one day. Understanding the position and power of the FDA and the AMA, I was now afraid to tell anyone else about the tea. These powerful organizations would never allow a beverage that cured colds and the flu in one day to be sold. They, and the pharmaceutical industry that they serve, had too much to lose. Fortunately for North Americans, my friends had no concept of the trouble they could get me into. Arizona was in the midst of a flu epidemic, and they told everyone they knew, "Jim May has leaves that will cure you in one day!" My phone rang day and night. But that's another story. Suffice it to say that I gave away all of the leaves I had on the condition that the people I gave them to tell me what happened. This would prove to be an important and wonderful experiment. Everyone—dozens of people, all suffering from the flu—were well in one day. They wanted more leaves, just to be prepared for the next time flu struck, and now I had none.

At that time I thought that the stevia leaves were used to give the tea its pleasantly sweet flavor and perhaps to mask the taste of the other two leaves. However, I was to learn that stevia leaves are extraordinarily healing themselves. Stevia, by itself, seems to help prevent colds and flu. And as I had amply observed, the blend of stevia, Amba-y, and Yaguarundi actually appeared to cure these conditions. At least, they left the person absolutely symptom free. Everyone felt completely well again. How the leaves worked, I didn't know. They apparently caused no adverse side effects, just healing. According to folklore, the Guarani had been using the beverage for about 2,000 years. I had now experienced the gentle power of this herbal tea myself. Thanks to dozens of fellow sufferers, I had both seen the results with my own eyes and heard them with my own ears. That was sufficient proof. I flew to Paraguay to learn more about these incredible leaves, which at the very least eliminated all of the symptoms of both colds and flu. In time this combination of prepared leaves would become known both in the United States and in Paraguay as Symfrë, (pronounced SIM free), a name suggested by my wife as a contraction of "symptom free."

HERBS THAT REJUVENATE BODY AND MIND

I arrived in Paraguay totally exhausted. Having had so much to do before my departure, I had not slept for the twenty-four hours prior to the flight, thinking I could sleep during the twenty-seven-hour trip. I was wrong. For the thirty-five years prior to that day I had suffered from severe allergies. We called it hay fever then. I was always allergic to nearly everything for which the doctors had tested me. Once, when the doctor had tested for twelve different substances by injecting them under the skin of my arm, I reacted to ten of them. My pincushioned arm turned red and swelled up like a balloon. I was miserable every day of my life, even though I took nearly every allergy medication and injection then known to medical science.

I am intensely allergic to tobacco smoke. It severely inhibits my ability to breathe. During the long flight from the United States to Paraguay, the plane was inundated with tobacco smoke. To save money, I had flown with a small Paraguayan airline. It did not have a nonsmoking section. Nearly everyone on the plane must have been smoking. It was awful! I tried holding a handkerchief over my mouth and nose to filter out the smoke but to no avail. I could not keep the smoke out of my nose and lungs. My bronchial tubes began to swell and become restricted. It felt as if my entire respiratory system was inflamed. Every breath was a struggle. What if I suffocated? I dared not sleep. I could not sleep. I huddled next to the window, keeping as low in the seat as possible, hoping that the smoke would rise above me. It was a horrible experience. I prayed silently just to survive the flight.

My young friend met me at the airport. He proudly announced that he had made appointments for me for virtually every hour of the day. We were to meet with farmers, businessmen, the press, and two members of the President's Cabinet, the Minister of Agriculture, and the Minister of Commerce. I told him that I was too sick and exhausted to see anyone. It had been more than forty-eight hours since I had slept, and I was miserable from my allergic reactions. I needed to sleep somewhere in clean fresh air. H. H. just looked at me and said, "I'll fix you some strong yerba maté. You'll be okay."

I looked at him in disbelief and responded, "You don't understand. I'm sick. I'm exhausted. I need to go to bed."

He smiled and said, "No, *you* don't understand. Just come with me. You'll be okay."

He took me to his apartment, where he began to pour, into two gourds, what I thought was a strange-looking, light greenish brown powdered substance with little pieces of twigs in it. He added crushed stevia leaves and filled the gourds with hot water, which caused the strange-looking brew to froth up on top. I could see the little twigs and other particles floating in the bubbly froth. He put a metal strawlike filtering device that he called a *bombilla* into each beverage. He then handed one gourd to me and began sipping the brew from the other as if it were the most delicious drink on earth. I looked at him in total disbelief. Did he really expect me to drink that gross-looking stuff?

"No thanks," I said as I handed the gourd back to him. "I don't know what this is. I'm not going to drink it."

"This is yerba maté with stevia," he responded. "It will help you. It will give you energy and make you feel better. We have a lot to do today. Trust me."

I gazed at the strange-looking brew for a moment, and then reasoned to myself that nothing could make me feel worse than I did already. My brain felt like mush. I could hardly produce a clear thought. My eyes were swollen, and I couldn't breathe through my nose. The leaves he sent me to cure colds and flu had worked astonishingly well. I took a small sip. The taste was different but not bad. In fact, it was pretty good. The stevia gave the drink a pleasant, sweet flavor. I continued to take small sips of the hot brew as we conversed.

Within fifteen to twenty minutes I realized that my brain had cleared. I was mentally alert and felt energized. I felt good! Was this a drug? Handing the remaining brew back to H. H., I told him, "I don't use drugs. I don't think I should drink this." I feared the leaves were really an illegal and potentially harmful drug.

He must have thought I was hopeless. "It's not a drug," he stated emphatically. "Yerba maté and stevia are pure nutrition. They are absolutely loaded with vitamins and minerals. They're just nourishing your body. That's why you feel so much energy."

I resisted. He persisted. He then told me the ancient Guarani legend of yerba maté.

THE LEGEND OF YERBA MATÉ

According to legend, the Guarani civilization began with two brothers who arrived in the distant past by ship, having sailed from a faraway land, crossing the great and vast ocean. The brothers vied for leadership, with the older brother, Tupi, constantly harassing and causing trouble for his younger brother, Guarani. Eventually, the hostilities became so severe that Guarani took his family, and those who wished to accompany them, and fled into the wilderness. In time they arrived at what is now Paraguay.

A variation of the story of the origin of the inhabitants of South America is that there was a large civilization living in the Caribbean area of Central America. They called themselves the "Caribe," meaning "The Saints." The brothers, who represented a fair-skinned people (the Guarani) and a darker-skinned people (the Tupi), left the settled land and traversed the great rivers of South America. They walked through the dense jungles and sailed upon many great rivers, eventually arriving in Paraguay, where they again feuded and divided into two separate factions. The Tupi became a fiercer, nomadic people and rejected the agricultural traditions of the Guarani. They discovered and drank a powerful caffeine-containing, highly addictive drink prepared from the Guaraná plant. The more stable Guarani people loved the land and became expert in agriculture and rain forest botany. They became excellent craftsmen in wood, stone, and precious metals. They were a deeply spiritual people who awaited the god whose coming to them had been foretold by their ancestors.

At this point the two versions of the story become identical. In time the tall, blue-eyed, fair-skinned, and bearded god Pá i Shume descended from the heavens wearing a flowing white robe and taught the people the principles of religion and more advanced concepts of agriculture. The most important agricultural technique he taught them was how to harvest, dry, cure, and prepare the leaves of a certain tree, from which they were to make a beverage. He told them that if they drank the beverage every day, it would ensure health, vitality, and longevity. Thus, the *yerba* (leaves) were harvested, cured, and ground into tiny pieces, which, along with a few of the broken twigs from the smaller leaf-laden branches, were placed in the *maté* (gourd). A little tepid water was added and then, after a few minutes, the maté was filled with steaming hot water and steeped for a few more minutes. It was then sipped through a *bombilla,* which was made of bamboo. Originally the drink was bitter, but when stevia, which at that time was called *ka'a eirete* (leaf-like-honey), was added, it became sweet and delicious. Now known as yerba maté, the beverage remains the most popular drink in all of South America. It is a powerful restorative and rejuvenator of health and well-being. It is believed that the fair-skinned god also taught the Guarani how to heal the body, through the many medicinal plants growing in their rain forests, and the spirit, through correct principles of worship and religion, now lost since the advent of the Europeans among them.

After hearing this intriguing legend, which had a familiar ring to it, I decided to finish my yerba maté and stevia beverage. In about forty-five minutes I suddenly realized that all of my horrible allergy symptoms were gone. They had completely vanished. I felt absolutely wonderful! I continued to drink this incredible, highly nourishing drink twice each day, as do the natives, and experienced no more allergic reactions during my entire stay in Paraguay. I was elated! But then, as I noted in my journal, maybe I just wasn't allergic to anything in Paraguay. However, since that day, I have learned about the healing secrets of yerba maté and other marvelous herbs of Paraguay. But that is another story for another time.

What a blessing it would be to all of mankind if Pá i Shume would descend again from heaven and teach the heads of the FDA and the AMA about the healing power of certain foods and herbs. Would these people comprehend the fact that certain plants are designed with the very nutrients, in their proper blend and balance, required by the glands and organs of the body to maintain a condition of health and vitality and to generate healing when necessary? In their arrogance and their ignorance of the gentle powers of nature, would they realize that, though their intentions might be good, they and the harsh drugs that they force upon us are the very causes of much of the suffering and death among human beings?

Some of the drugs made by man have their time and place, and can relieve pain and suffering. Like herbs, they should be used with wisdom and skill, but never merely to make a profit or for the convenience of the physician. Some medical drugs, like the healing plants of nature, can be used daily to nourish and aid certain glands and organs, and to assist the body in its normal functions. Some should be used only for short periods of time, to support the body until it recovers and regains its own ability to produce the needed chemicals in their proper balance. Others are too harsh and destructive, only masking the symptoms while exacerbating the real problem, and should never have been approved. The side effects—the destructive influences they cause within the body—are often worse than the disease or condition for which they were prescribed.

You see many such drugs advertised daily on television. But did you know that some of these drugs, so heavily promoted, were neither developed nor approved for the use, disease, or condition for which they are being advertised and sold? I believe it is a marketing ploy allowed by the FDA to extend the life of a patent and thus to significantly increase profits. You didn't know? Well, now you know. What man will do for money is shameful.

I wonder. Should the Master Physician come again, would the FDA and AMA require Him to exchange His flowing white celestial robe for a white duster and stethoscope before they listen to him? Would they require Him to attend medical school before permitting Him to teach us about the healing plants of His creation and how they affect the human body? Perhaps they, too, are among the learned of our times who the Apostle Paul so aptly described when he wrote, "Ever learning but never able to come to a knowledge of the truth" (2 Timothy 3:7).

Prayers and wishes aside, I could not learn about these remarkable herbs fast enough. There was neither question nor doubt in my mind. I wanted to bring these incredibly healing herbs of Paraguay to the United States. But how could we do this? Where should we start? We began to discuss the possibilities. When H. H. told me that yerba maté was on the FDA's GRAS list, the decision was made. Yerba maté would not pose a problem with the FDA. I did not think that North Americans would be very excited about drinking the loose form, with all of its floating particles, through a *bombilla,* so we set out to find a tea-bagging machine. There were two in all of Paraguay. We were finally able to arrange for time on one of them to make tea bags of yerba maté, as well as of a blend of yerba maté and stevia that we would call YerbaMaté Royale. However, it would be several months before the time on the tea-bagging machine became available to us. I would make my second journey to Paraguay before that time came around.

For some reason that I did not understand at the time, I was concerned about using the name *stevia* on the packaging that had to be designed and printed. With a little research we discovered the ancient Guarani name *ka'a eirete*. That was the perfect name for this unique leaf. Later, I registered the name *HoneyLeaf* in Paraguay as a legal trademark. Time proved this inspiration to be a true blessing. When the FDA placed a total ban on stevia, no one questioned the ingredient named honeyleaf that was a part of an ancient Guarani Indian herbal blend, which it was. The word *sweet*, however, could not appear on the packaging. When FDA or customs inspectors inquired about honeyleaf, I truthfully replied that it was a commonly used Paraguayan herb and had been a part of the YerbaMaté Royale blend for centuries.

With my second trip to Paraguay in mid-1983, my intrigue with stevia and the other incredible healing herbs of Paraguay changed to excitement. I began telling everyone about these herbs and giving samples to relatives and friends, including medical doctors. All of these people, including the physicians, related wonderful stories of healing that they attributed to the Paraguayan herbs. They were all astounded with the results they achieved and wanted more herbs. It was a heart surgeon who both encouraged and motivated me to forget about returning to the dialysis program and instead concentrate my attention on getting the herbs to Americans. My family and friends wanted more herbs and, more importantly, I wanted knowledge. The herbs I could order with ease, but finding reliable information was a totally different matter. My personal program of research into these specific plants commenced in earnest and continues to this day.

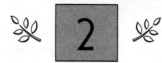

From the Rain Forests of Paraguay to the Kitchens of the World

"When one first observes the plant, nothing particular about it summons the attention, but when even a small piece of the leaf is placed in the mouth, one is amazed by its sweetness. A mere fragment of the leaf is enough to sweeten the mouth for an hour."

—Dr. Moisés S. Bertoni (1857–1929),
discoverer of stevia in modern times

The use of stevia for improving the flavor of food and drinks began centuries ago, around the campfires of the Guarani living in the rain forests of Paraguay. As these people discovered stevia's numerous and miraculous healing properties, they began to prize it as a virtual sacred treasure.

During the past century, scientists worldwide have become fascinated with this unique plant and its incredible potential. By 2002, more than a thousand scientific studies and patents were published. In the not-too-distant future, I expect consumers throughout the world will have learned about the many preventative and restorative benefits of stevia. When that day arrives, I believe stevia will become a staple in the kitchens of the world for its nutritional and health-generating properties, as well as for its sweetening ability. Wise consumers will keep whole-leaf forms of stevia in their medicine cabinets and first-aid kits because of its unique ability to reduce pain, stop sore throats, inhibit the growth of oral bacteria, and heal minor wounds rapidly while leaving no scars. The more you learn about the healing qualities of this remarkable leaf, the more convinced you will become that stevia truly is a miracle plant.

WHAT IS STEVIA?

Stevia rebaudiana Bertoni is a unique and potentially revolutionary plant that is native to the areas near the rain forests of northeastern Paraguay, where it grows in groupings of two or three small shrubs. Its natural habitat is on the edges of marshes and grasslands in relatively infertile, acidic sands or muck, with shallow water tables. Paraguayan professors of botany believe it has been in constant use by the natives of this area for more than 1,500 years. In the beginning the natives used it to freshen the mouth and to sweeten and mellow the strong taste of yerba maté as well as other herbal preparations. No one knows when its unique medicinal qualities were first discovered but this, too, must have been in antiquity. It is reported that in the pre-Columbian era the Paraguayan people used stevia to sweeten alcoholic beverages and to improve the taste of tobacco. They also prepared small capsules that the tribal herbalist or medicine man would give to anyone experiencing either physical or emotional fatigue or what we now know to be diabetes. These early Paraguayans quickly learned about its tonic action on the stomach.[1] A few leaves in hot water will provide relief to an upset stomach in minutes.

It would not have taken much experimentation for the ancients to learn that by cooking the leaves in water, a dark brownish, intensely sweet, highly concentrated and thickened, licorice-flavored, powerful healing agent was released. They would have soon realized that under certain conditions of listlessness, lethargy, and dizziness, ingesting this liquid restores energy and mental alertness. They would have learned that in this easy-to-apply liquid form, it could also heal nearly any kind of cut or sore on the body or lips, or within the mouth, and had a "shelf life" of years. They would also have discovered the effectiveness of the dark, syruplike liquid in healing numerous skin problems, as well as softening the skin and reducing wrinkles.

The current Guarani name for stevia is *ka'a he'e,* meaning "sweet leaf" or "sweet herb." In other native languages it is *azuca-ca'a* or *ca'a-e'h e.* These names for stevia describe its sweet, nectarlike flavor. The tribal name *azuca-ca'a* gives credibility to the story that Spanish settlers, who came to Paraguay in the early 1500s, also used the leaf as a sweetener. *Azúcar* is Spanish for "sugar." While it cannot be proven from existing records, it is believed—and completely logical—that these early Spaniards sent stevia leaves back to Spain. Having "discovered" this unique *azuca-ca'a* (sugar leaf) among the Guarani, they undoubtedly sent samples of the sweet, sugarlike leaves from Paraguay to the Spanish Royalty and the hierarchy of the Catholic Church.

Had the Spanish settlers been able to solve the unique problems of the large-scale cultivation of stevia at that time in history, perhaps stevia would have been in widespread use throughout Europe before the commencement of the seventeenth century. One can only imagine the difference this would have made in the dietary habits of Europeans and, eventually, Americans. Had this occurred, stevia might well have been one of the cherished plants brought to America by the Pilgrims, who then could have introduced it to the Native Americans, completing the circle.

It is believed that owing to the difficulties with finding wild stevia plants in the rain forest and with learning to domesticate and cultivate the plants, honey became the primary sweetener for the earliest natives of northeastern Paraguay. This helps us to understand why the ancients called stevia *ka'a eirete,* or "leaf-like-honey." Some Paraguayans still refer to the water-based, concentrated stevia preparation as "stevia honey."

As a matter of fact, I was not totally convinced concerning the natural sweetness of stevia until May 1983, when I journeyed to northeastern Paraguay, walked into a stevia field, picked a leaf from a plant, and placed it in my mouth. It was the same delicately sweet, delightfully refreshing, honeylike flavor that I had first experienced months earlier.

Since the Spanish did not commercially export large quantities of stevia to Spain, as the Jesuit priests did yerba maté, it is evident that the problems with cultivating stevia had not yet been mastered. In time it was learned that the seeds rapidly become infertile but that stevia can be cultivated from cuttings from mother plants. Soon small farms began to emerge in northeastern Paraguay and in the contiguous areas of Brazil and Argentina, where it is now grown commercially.

At maturity, stevia is a small shrub, growing to a height of two and a half to three feet. It is an herb of the *Compositae* (daisy) family, producing small white blossoms at the terminal of the stems and arranged in panicles. The fruit or seed is an achene, so it ripens without bursting its sheath. The seeds are centered within tiny, curved, stick-like fibers in the shape of a parasol. They, therefore, are dispersed by the slightest movement of the air, whether caused by the wind or the passing of a human, an animal, or a bird. The sweetness of the small, lanceolated, obtuse leaves depends on the hours of sunlight shining on the plant. The longer the day and the brighter the sun, the sweeter the leaf.

The plant is delicate and requires tender, loving care from the moment the seed is placed upon, or the cutting is planted within, the soil to the day of harvest. Proper temperatures, humidity, cultivation methods, and frequency of irrigation are critical to its survival. While it is grown successfully in other parts of the world, this botanical wonder does best in the warm, humid climate of the subtropics. Many people have attempted to grow stevia in their home gardens or as an indoor plant. However, while growing stevia at home may be fun to try, it may be too difficult for the novice gardener and will rarely produce high-quality leaves. Nevertheless, stevia plants can now be purchased at plant nurseries throughout America. It is fun to grow a plant in the kitchen and a delightful experience to place a stevia leaf upon the tongue and enjoy the delicate sweet taste of excellent nutrition.

While living plants and seeds have been exported from Paraguay and stevia is now grown commercially in many countries, no foreign leaves have as yet measured up to the quality and taste of the South American–grown leaves. Exceptions to this come from the plants grown in some small experimental fields, under the watchful eye of skilled agronomists, for the research and development of higher-glycoside-yielding varieties. Glycosides, as mentioned in

Chapter 1, are the compounds within stevia leaves that give them their delicately sweet taste. While the glycosides are from 250 to 400 times sweeter than sugar, a good-quality stevia leaf is about 30 times sweeter than common sugar. What makes stevia so appealing as a sweetener is that scientific research has aptly demonstrated that the human body does not digest or metabolize these intensely sweet glycosides. They pass unchanged through the entire alimentary canal (from the mouth to the elimination orifice) without being assimilated into the body. Therefore, we obtain no calories from pure stevia in any of its consumable forms and it has a glycemic index of zero.

The greatest volume of stevia is currently produced in China, but at least to this date, the leaves are not as sweet as those grown in South America. It is unclear why this is so. Perhaps it has to do with the pollution in China's air and water, or within its soil, which has been overrun and farmed for millennia and thus lacks vital nutrients. Or it may be the climate. The virgin lands surrounding the rain forests of South America are different from China. Where stevia grows best, the undisturbed and easily drained unpolluted soil is naturally moist but not drenched, nor is it overly fertile. The air is pure, the soil and water unpolluted, and the sun-laden days are long and humid.

To the dismay of modern farmers attempting to capitalize on the recent demand for stevia leaves, once the plant blossoms, the sweetness of its leaves significantly diminishes. Therefore, the window of opportunity for harvesting maximum quality stevia leaves is narrow. The farmer must choose between producing quality leaves or harvesting seeds.

STEVIA BECOMES KNOWN TO THE WORLD OF RESEARCH

The commercial possibilities of stevia were recognized in the last decade of the 1800s. Having first heard of the plant in 1887 and receiving his first samples a few years later, Dr. Moisés Santiago Bertoni, director of the College of Agriculture in Asunción, Paraguay, published the first known description of stevia in *Revista de Agronomía* in 1899. At that time he named the plant *Eupatorium*

Rebaudianum, to honor the Paraguayan chemist Dr. Ovidio Rebaudi, who in 1900 received a specimen from Dr. Bertoni and made what was then considered to be the first "complete" chemical study of stevia leaves.

Dr. Rebaudi proved that the chemical in stevia that gives it the flavor and aroma of licorice is not the same as that found in the root of the licorice plant. He was also the first modern scientist to discover and separate an aromatic resin from stevia containing a bitter element that he recognized to have an application in medicine. Though the chemistry of the resin was not completely understood at that time, Dr. Rebaudi believed it would have special benefits for stomach and digestive problems. He was correct. He published his research in *Revista de Quimica y Farmacia* in 1900.

In 1901, Cecil Gosling, the British consul at Asunción, sent a sample of stevia leaves along with Bertoni's description to the Kew Botanical Gardens, near London. In describing the sweet taste of stevia, Gosling said that "a few leaves of this sweet herb are sufficient to sweeten a strong cup of coffee or tea, giving it also a pleasant aromatic flavor."[2]

Commercial agricultural projects commenced in 1902, and by 1908 Paraguayan farmers were harvesting one ton per hectare (2.47 acres). With the new advances in farming techniques, the use of stevia increased substantially among the general population. It is currently estimated that over the past century, many stevia users have consumed as much as 5 to 10 grams per day in their hot yerba maté or coffee.[3] This is a very substantial amount of stevia. No one has ever reported any harm resulting from the continuous ingestion of such large amounts of stevia on a daily basis.

In Germany, P. Rasenack first isolated the sweet principle, then called a glucoside, in crystalline form in 1908.[4] His research was followed by Karl Dietrich, who published his chemical analysis of stevia in *Chemische Zeitung* in 1909. In 1913, research of the "now famous stevia" continued in laboratories in Antwerp, Wiesbaden, and Hamburg. As more research was conducted, it became apparent that the plant had been inappropriately classified. Bertoni redefined it as *Stevia rebaudiana*, a member of the *Compositae* family. Finally, it became known as *Stevia rebaudiana Bertoni*, to pay well-deserved homage to the two doctors responsible for bringing the world the first knowledge of this incredible miracle of nature. The genus *Stevia* is named after Peter James Esteve, a Spanish professor of botany who died in 1566.

Many writers have improperly instructed their readers to pronounce "stevia" as STEE vee uh. This is not correct. Doctor Esteve was Spanish. In the Spanish language, the "e" is pronounced more like the long "a" in the English words "may" or "lay." But even the Spanish-speaking South Americans often pronounce the "e" as in the English word "met."

I take it as a sincere compliment when people ask me, "Did you name stee-vee-uh after your son Steve?" But such is not the case, nor the correct pronunciation. Apparently, we North Americans want to Americanize everything. Just remember that all three names are from the Spanish and Latin languages, where "i" is pronounced like the English "y," with the sound of ee, and "a" is pronounced like ah. Thus, STE vee ah or STAY vee ah. The scientific and, therefore, Latin name is actually taken from Spanish: *Stevia rebaudiana Bertoni.* Steve, however, counsels me to give up and go with the flow. "People in America call it stee-vee-uh and you are not going to change them." Where have the times gone when we ancients had influence upon the young?

In 1915, R. Kobert lectured in Europe on the "Sweet principles of Eupatorium and Glycyrhiza," and in 1920, the *Bulletin of the Imperial Institute* included an article titled "The Cá a-êhê Plant as a Sweetening Agent."[5] One of Dr. Bertoni's next articles on stevia was titled "Stevina and Rebaudiana: New Sweetening Substances." It was published in *Anales Científicos Paraguayos* in 1918, and in it Dr. Bertoni referred to the German research. This document is on file in the U.S. Department of Agriculture (USDA) Library. In this report Dr. Bertoni quoted from *The Official Public Laboratory of Hamburg,* which stated: "The specimens received are of the well known plant which alarmed sugar producers some years ago. The sweet substance contained in the leaves is about 180 times as sweet as cane-sugar. . . . The plant does not have an equal in the potency of its saccharines, but in its industrial application it probably cannot enter into competition with the known kinds of sugar-cane and beet sugars—being limited to medicinal uses for the preparation of saccharine for diabetics." Dr. Bertoni then suggested, "The principle importance of Ka'a He'e is due to the possibility of substituting it for saccharine. It presents these great advantages over saccharine:

1. It is not toxic but, on the contrary, it is healthful, as shown by *long experience* and according to the studies of Dr. Rebaudi.

2. It is a sweetening agent of great power.

3. It can be employed directly in its natural state (pulverized leaves).

4. It is much cheaper than saccharine."

He then makes this revealing statement, considering the current position of the FDA that stevia was unknown before 1958, except by a small group of Guarani natives: "Small specimens sent by me to Europe and North America awakened lively interest, even enthusiasm, invariably bringing forth orders which ranged in size from kilos to tons. The advantages which the plant presents—that over sugar for various medicinal uses (syrups, liquors, diabetic, etc.) . . . the enormous sweetening power . . . and the agreeable flavor of the syrup or liquor prepared with it—prove not excessive the optimism in expecting a smiling future for Stevina."[6] A metric ton is 1,000 kilos, or 2,200 pounds. It takes an enormous amount of stevia leaves to weigh a metric ton.

In 1921, at a meeting of the Union Internationale de Chimie, held in Copenhagan, Denmark, "stevioside" was adopted as the name for the crystalline glucoside of *Stevia rebaudiana*. Interest in stevia now expanded rapidly, with the French chemists M. Bridel and R. Lavieille making a detailed examination of stevia and publishing a series of reports in 1931. They also reported on the safety of stevia in the guinea pig, rabbit, and rooster.[7] That same year researcher M. Pomaret joined Lavieille to demonstrate that stevioside is excreted mostly without structural modification.[8] Their studies are still quoted extensively in the scientific literature. In 1937, E. Thomas added to the rapidly increasing sphere of knowledge concerning the properties of stevia. He gave the sweetening power of stevioside as 300 times that of sucrose and outlined the best conditions for growing *Stevia rebaudiana Bertoni*.

Even with this compelling research, there was no strong demand in Europe or the United States for a sugar replacement. We were not yet aware of how harmful refined sugar is to the human body. Once again Paraguayan interest in growing stevia waned. However, with the outbreak of World War II and the reduction in the availability resulting in the rationing of sugar, authorities in Great Britain began to look for a substitute. In 1941, a Dr. Meiville prepared a glowing memorandum about *Stevia rebaudiana* for the director of the Royale Botanic Gardens, in which he presented the possibility of cultivating stevia in Britain as a substitute for imported cane sugar. He suggested methods of agriculture that would enable stevia to be grown in Britain. Among them, he suggested glass "greenhouses." A similar strategy had been adopted by Napoleon during the British blockade of France and led to the establishment of the sugar beet industry in France.[9]

The process for extracting sugar from beets had been developed in Germany in 1747 by Andreas Marggrat. By the first decade of the 1800s, Great Britain ruled the seas, including the Caribbean, and controlled the sugar-cane trade. Napoleon feared that France's sugar supply from the Caribbean cane fields would be blockaded by the British in their continuing dispute with the newly proclaimed nation of the United States of America. This British blockade was one of the major issues that led to the War of 1812. Thus, in 1811 Napoleon ordered hundreds of beet processing factories to be built in France. Farmers purchased their beet stock from Germany. When Napoleon fell from power, the young industry collapsed. In those days, sugar beets contained only about 2 percent sugar. Over the years, sugar beet varieties have been bred to contain 17 to 18 percent sugar.[10]

The original Paraguayan stevia plants contained 9 to 12 percent sweet glycosides and have recently been bred to contain 28 to 30 percent glycosides. Is it any wonder that Dr. Meiville suggested stevia as the answer to the shortage of sugar in Great Britain during World War II?

Why not produce stevia sugar in Great Britain? As he discussed in his book *Stevia Rebaudiana: Nature's Sweet Secret* (Vital Health Publishing, 1999), David Richard found that "newspaper articles [of that time] reported that these experiments were successful in Cornwall and Devon, where the equivalent of two tons of sugar per acre were shown to be possible to produce. However, for some unknown reason, the project was set aside."

The lumbering wheels of government progress slowly, and the war ended before the necessary agricultural and extraction facilities could be developed and put into production. Had the project materialized, we would be sweetening our food and drink with stevia and not sugar, saccharine, or aspartame derivatives. The world would be a much more healthful place in which to live, with a significantly reduced number of people suffering from obesity, diabetes, hypoglycemia, and the other sugar/aspartame-related diseases. You could be enjoying healthful and low-calorie candy, chewing gum, soft drinks, ice cream, pies, and cakes, without concern for weight gain or sugar/aspartame-related health problems. Can you imagine the pleasure of eating your favorite candy or ice cream without worrying about weight gain or tooth decay? Where were the French and Lafayette when the Americans really needed them?

A much more detailed report on stevia was prepared in 1945 by L. A. Gattoni, and submitted to the Medical Plants Division of the Instituto Agronomico Nacional de Paraguay. He advocated the establishment of a stevioside industry in Paraguay as part of the national drive to export products from Paraguay. He believed that stevioside would become an advantageous replacement for saccharine. He even outlined a process for the commercial production of stevioside, or a stevia concentrate, and provided a detailed cost estimate. Gattoni was convinced that such a project would be commercially profitable.[11]

Unfortunately for the Paraguayan economy, nothing was done to put the project into action. Perhaps the wheels of the Paraguayan government were bogged down in the deep muck resulting from the annual flooding of the Parana River. In addition, there was great demand for cotton and beef, which seemed to be more viable industries. After all, a steak on the plate is better than two leaves in the bush. Also, Paraguay's economy was ill prepared to suppport an extensive and expensive new industry in the agriculture and processing technology required for producing and marketing stevioside to the world.

At about this same time, in the United States, the National Institutes of Health (NIH) attempted to grow stevia. Certainly we Americans could achieve success where the British had failed. Alas, the seeds, which had probably been stored for months or even years, would not germinate. The project was abandoned with the comment that stevia was nothing more than a "botanical curiosity." It was unworthy of the NIH's continued interest. Ignorance is bliss. These "brilliant minds" had not bothered to do their homework and learn what the uneducated Paraguayan farmers already knew about planting and growing stevia.

Man needed to wait a few more decades to receive the special gift that is stevia. Besides, Hawaii needed to grow sugarcane, and the sugar beet industry was growing rapidly and filling the demand in America. However, during the early 1950s a scientific branch of the U.S. Public Health Service based in Bethesda, Maryland, published its research on stevia. For the first time ion exchange had been utilized to obtain nearly pure stevioside. The research confirmed the intense sweetness and the molecular structure determined by Bridel and Lavielle in 1931.

For the Japanese, the situation was different. In the mid-1950s Japanese farmers needed substitute crops for rice. With the end of the war, and the Americanization of Japan, demand for rice was plummeting. Apparently, being smarter, or at least thinking more clearly than the Americans, the Japanese did not want to create enormous surpluses of rice by establishing artificial price supports for rice farmers. They set out to find alternative crops.

Being 100 percent net importers of sugar, the Japanese found the idea of creating an internal source of an alternative sweetener to be compelling. Not only would they give their farmers another cash crop, but they would also create new industries to process the leaves into stevioside and to market the stevioside to food processors. This was a win-win situation, they felt. Stevioside lacked the bulking and browning properties of sugar, but these were considered minimal problems that could be resolved. If Napoleon and the French could establish a sugarbeet industry, certainly the Japanese could be successful with stevia. Even if they could not defeat the Americans or British in war, they could beat them in the competition to develop the safest and most healthful sweetener ever discovered by man.

While We Were Sleeping

While the Americans and the British—and the Paraguayans— slept through the time for action, the Japanese put their plan into operation. In 1954 the Japanese Ministry of Agriculture began to organize for the agricultural production of stevia, initially in Paraguay. Not only were the Paraguayans encouraged to grow stevia, but Japanese farmers now living in Paraguay also established stevia farms. Not seeing, or at least not being able to read, the writing on the wall in Japanese characters, the Paraguayan farmers were jubilant. They had a market for their stevia. Every farmer in Paraguay now wanted to grow stevia and get rich off the Japanese. Phase one of the battle strategy was under way.

Phase two commenced in 1956 when the Japanese government provided the needed resources for the toxicological evaluation of stevia. This research commenced under the direction of Professor Hiroshi Mitsuhashi at Hokkaido University. Unknown to the common farmers in Paraguay, the Japanese were quietly taking stevia seeds and plant seedlings to Japan. Next, the Japanese authorities selected about fifty areas suitable for growing stevia—in the warm, temperate, and subtropical regions of southern Japan in Kyushu as well as in the surrounding Asian countries of Taiwan, Malaysia, Indonesia, Singapore, and South Korea. By 1984, Hank Dom, an American who had been living in Indonesia cultivating rubber trees, came to me with a proposal to establish stevia plantations there and compete with the Japanese. But it was too soon and I possessed no funds for such a project. Clearly, this was a blessing in disguise considering the current problems in Indonesia.

Following the work of the Bethesda scientists in the 1950s and the development of thin layer chromatography and gas liquid chromatography, Japanese university and corporate scientists were able to develop and patent new, more efficient methods of identifying, extracting, and separating the various sweet glycosides from stevia leaves. The required research to prove the safety of stevia and its glycosides as sweeteners followed rapidly. Japanese scientists studied both acute toxicity and subacute toxicity of stevia crude extract, refined extract, and crude crystals. They reported no harmful effects from eating large amounts of stevia. Gladys Planas, a chemist with the University of the Republic, Montevideo, Uruguay, and Joseph Kuc, a biochemist with Purdue University, Lafayette, Indiana, in 1968 had reported that stevia was a natural contraceptive, and the Japanese scientists tried repeatedly but without success to duplicate the results. (For a full discussion of the Planas-Kuc research, see Chapter 7.) Continued research conducted by the General Safety Research Institute and the Food and Drug Safety Center established that stevia was *not* a natural contraceptive, was *not* carcinogenic, and did *not* cause mutations. In fact, the Japanese scientists declared that stevia offered numerous health benefits to humans and predicted that "stevia will become [a] major natural sweetener in the future."[12] They said that stevia is appropriate for use in food and drinks of all kinds, including carbonated beverages, orange juice, chewing gum, frozen deserts, ice cream, sherbets, fish pasta, salt pickles, bean paste, soy sauce, and all sorts of low-calorie foods.

The data coming from the science laboratories of Japan, combined with the previous research from Europe, the United States, and South America as well as the evidence of centuries of safe use in Paraguay, was sufficient. Completely satisfied, the Japanese Ministry of Health and Welfare accepted the validity of the research and approved the new sweetener for use in both foods and beverages.[13] Stevia has now been in constant use in Japan as a commercial sweetener for more than thirty years. No contraceptive effect or harm of any kind to humans has been reported.

At this point we must pause in the narrative to emphasize an important point of fact—and to pose a question. Do you remember why the FDA refused to allow stevia to be grandfathered under the GRAS classification? It insisted that stevia was a rare and unknown plant, except to a small group of Guarani Indians, prior to 1958. Yet all of the facts just presented were contained in the research documents given to the FDA in the two petitions presented by the Lipton Tea Company and the AHPA. Apparently, and unfortunately, it appears that neither of these petitioners had studied the scientific data sufficiently to comprehend it and then organize it into a logical and informative format for presentation. The question must be asked: Had the petitions been better prepared and the data correctly arranged and verified by scientists, would the FDA have studied the data and approved stevia as GRAS? Would obesity, diabetes, and tooth decay be among the major health problems facing Americans today?

Until the mid-1970s, the unsuspecting native and Japanese farmers in Paraguay continued to prosper and export their leaves to Japan. By this time production in the Orient was sufficient to meet the demand in Japan and the farmers in Paraguay were cut off without warning. The "S-bomb" was dropped. With no market for their stevia leaves, the farmers lost everything. Totally dejected, they either attempted to grow other crops or just quit farming. Among the Paraguayans, interest in stevia again waned.

During this period of time, Hernando Bertoni, a grandson of Moisés Bertoni, held the position of Minister of Agriculture in Paraguay. I had the privilege of meeting with Dr. Bertoni during my first visit there in 1983. It was a most pleasant experience. I presented my plans for introducing stevia into the United States, as a replacement for sugar. He expressed his hopes that stevia's day was finally arriving and pledged his complete cooperation. Unknown to either of us, however, the storm clouds of opposition were again forming in the United States. In those early days I was as naïve as the Paraguayan farmers. Fortunately, naïveté is often the forerunner of progress. Without it, many of the advancements mankind now enjoys would have never been attempted by the dreamers and visionaries who first thought of them.

In 1983, I imported the first of my Paraguayan products into the United States as a commercial venture. These products included YerbaMaté, YerbaMaté Royale (with stevia), Symfrë (also with stevia), and Nectar of HoneyLeaf (pure stevia concentrate), which I gave away. People were so enthusiastic about the results they were experiencing that I began to sell the shelf-ready, packaged herbs out of my garage. I had no concept of what lay in store for me, not realizing that I was walking on quicksand. It would be three years before the enterprise would net a dime. In fact, my wife and I would have to sell everything we owned except our home and auto to make ends meet and to keep the fledgling herbal products business, Wisdom of the Ancients, from sinking into the mire. We had lost far more than our original investment. By the end of the fourth year I was finally able to take a small income, which totaled $16,000. Everything else was gone. Well-meaning friends, family, and neighbors ridiculed and chastised me. Numerous times I was admonished, "Stop this foolishness and get a job!" College professors counseled my wife to get rid of her ignorant husband. But my course was fixed. I knew the truth. I knew that Americans needed stevia and the other healing herbs of Paraguay. These incredible herbs would make a profound difference in their health and well-being.

Besides all of this, the NutraSweet people, at that time the G.D. Searle Company, were soon to hear of me. The October 1985 issue of *Vegetarian Times* magazine printed a couple of short paragraphs about the blessings and health benefits of Wisdom of the Ancients stevia concentrate. The quicksand would soon open its mouth to swallow and suffocate me. (See Chapter 13.)

Interest continued in the United States, however. The University of California at Davis began an experimental project to grow stevia. Clinton C. Shock, research assistant in the Department of Agronomy and Range Science, was dispatched to Paraguay to study stevia. He collected seeds and live plants in the wild, along the tributaries of the Ypané River in Northeastern Paraguay. Upon his return, seeds were planted in the university's greenhouse and at its experimental farm. Germination was poor, but by 1979 the researchers had about 200 stevia plants to set out in the fields. The project continued for a few years.[14,15] Shock, who had learned much about propagating stevia under domestic conditions, eventually left the university. In 1996, a few years after reading his research, I wanted to talk with him. My sleuthing efforts paid off and I was able to locate him. We had a fascinating conversation. His interest in stevia and its commercial potential remained high. He, too, believed in the future of stevia, and was delighted that someone had "picked up the ball" and was running with it.

In 1985, following an interview on a Denver radio station about the healing herbs of Paraguay, I was informed of an enterprise in Colorado to grow and sell stevia. The Stevia Company was growing fields of stevia in a commercial venture for which it was selling shares to the general public. After returning to Phoenix, I was contacted by a securities company that was handling the placement of the stock and given the company's prospectus. I held back my amusement until after I had left the investment counselor. Stevia plants cannot survive the slightest frost, let alone the freezing temperatures of a Colorado winter. At best, the company would get one crop per year. Each spring it would have the costly problem of planting low-germinating seeds in a greenhouse, which would then need to be transplanted to fields, where they would grow to maturity during a short summer. I informed the investment counselor of these agricultural facts and suggested that the project was doomed and the investors would lose their money. However, I was to learn at a later time that this company had been involved in considerable research in both agricultural and extraction methodology. It was trying to develop a strain of stevia that would be more resistant to frost. Unfortunately, by this time the FDA had become determined to remove stevia from the kitchens of America. With no market for stevia leaves or extract, and no real solution to the frost problem, the company soon went bankrupt.

However, research continued in California, Japan, South Korea, Thailand, China, Brazil, Canada, and Israel. An agricultural project was even being conducted in the semiarid region on the borders of the Negev Desert.[16] Some of us were already well aware that stevia cannot survive in a hot, dry climate. Stevia must have continuous moisture, a humid climate, and well-drained soil.

In 1983, before I began importing any herbal products, I took the products to the FDA office in Phoenix. I wanted an approval before going to the expense of packaging and bringing the Paraguayan herbs to the United States. Each time I brought a product in, I was assured that there was no problem. When I brought in my Nectar of HoneyLeaf, I suggested the agency take the whole-leaf stevia concentrate and examine it, send it to its own lab, or do whatever it desired. The reply was, "We know about stevia. It's okay. As long as we get no consumer complaints about your product, you have no problem." Famous last words! To read what happened, see Chapter 13.

Why does stevia stir such controversy, fear, and reprisal from the pharmaceutical, medical, and artificial sweetener establishments? The next three chapters will help you to better understand their fear of stevia. In these chapters, we will learn about the incredible healing qualities of stevia. The different forms of stevia offer varying degrees of benefits. It is important to understand them all in order to make informed decisions concerning which stevia products are appropriate for you and your family. In Chapter 10 we will then return to the fascinating story of how the FDA/artificial-sweetener opposition was finally overcome and stevia became available to the citizens of America.

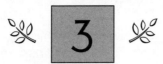

3

Healing the Body with Sweetness and Wisdom: Whole-Leaf Stevia

"What a piece of work is man! How noble in reason! How infinite in faculty! In form, in moving, how express and admirable! In action how like an angel! In apprehension how like a god!"

—From *Hamlet* by William Shakespeare (1564–1616)

Since the passage of the Dietary Supplement Health and Education Act of 1994, stevia has gained rapid popularity among health-conscious Americans, holistic physicians, and nutritionists. However, because much has been written about stevia by people who really do not understand the various consumable forms of the herb nor their sweetness equivalents as compared to sugar, many people are confused. The consumer has not been adequately informed about which form of stevia is best for his or her specific need or desire. The intent of this book is to give you accurate information about every form of consumable stevia available as of this writing. Each form of stevia will be discussed first for its ability to heal, and then also for its uses as a sweetener or to enhance flavor. When you finish reading this chapter and the next two, you will appreciate the miracle of nature that is stevia.

NUTRIENTS, PHYTOCHEMICALS, AND A WELL-ORCHESTRATED YOU

Herbalists teach that certain herbs heal the body. I suggest that Pavvo Airola, Ph.D., a noted healer, author and herbalist, was more correct when he wrote that herbs are healing agents, that is, they provide the stimulus, the nutrients and the phytochemicals, in correct combination and balance, required for the healing of the body. The human body is endowed with incredible capabilities, including the ability to correct its inner processes and to heal its own several parts. This healing happens in and of itself, without your constant, conscious awareness. There are, however, certain requirements that you must consciously fulfill:

- You must provide your body with the full complement of required nutrients and fibers contained within the various natural foods and herbs.

- You must treat your body (including your brain) with wisdom and respect, demanding neither too little nor too much of it and its several organs, glands, tissues, and cells.

- You must honor your body by keeping it free of substances that are harmful or toxic, which destroy cells, interrupt rhythms, interfere with impulses, and reduce communication between the cells, between the brain and the mind, and between the body and the spirit.

- You must activate and energize your body with the power of your mind (conscious thought or faith) to control and to heal.

When you fail to do the above, you have no promise of health or well-being. When you neglect or abuse your body (including your brain) with harmful substances, it cannot respond in the manner in which it was designed.

Your body is a remarkable feat of physical, chemical, magnetic, electrical, and energy engineering. Each part of this highly complex system depends upon accurate input from the other parts. The processes of communication and response between your spirit mind, physical brain, emotions, and each gland, organ, tissue, cell, atom, and subparticle are miraculous. All of the "strings" of the physical instrument that is you must play with precision and in beautiful harmony if you wish to make your total being a symphony of life, with lovely, soul-pleasing, and recurring melodic refrains.

We each possess a physical instrument that is unique in and of itself. None of our instruments is *exactly* like any others. No one else on earth has, or ever has had, or ever will have, a body that is precisely like yours. The exact pitch, range, and quality of tone that you add to the "grand harmonic symphony of life" cannot be produced by any other being in this or any generation of time. It is true that the quality of your personal instrument is greatly influenced by the purity of the materials used to create it. These basic materials were provided through your ancestral genetic code or genome. We carry within our cellular structure the pleasing tones produced by chords playing in harmony as well as the brash tones produced by dissonant sounds. However, we also have the abilities to cleanse our personal instrument and give it tender loving care, thus enhancing its tonal quality and bringing it into perfect intonation with the grand symphony of life. We can also ensure that the instruments that issue forth from our own reproductive processes will be composed of materials that are pure and, thus, are able to produce tones that will bring solace to the heart and joy to the soul, in the concert of their lives. Then, as we look upon our posterity and reflect back upon the refrain of our own creation, we, too, will have joy.

Keep Your Body in Tune with Its Own Inner Self

You have two great maestros of your total being: your mind and your brain. Your brain is the grand conductor of your body, in all of its functions and physical expressions. Your mind is the maestro of your brain. Your brain is the willing and obedient servant of your mind. It will strive to obey the thoughts you place and hold in focus within it. It will strive to produce the melody and the harmonies created within your mind, whether the result is beautiful and soothing or shocking and disharmonic. Your brain, however, cannot conduct the symphony of life composed within your own mind unless all of the members of your personal orchestra are in tune with each other and ready to produce their own specific and unique tones with beauty and precision. The orchestra of your total body must be well nourished. It must be energized both physically and mentally. To produce the harmonic and beautiful symphonies of life, it must receive all of the nutrients that are essential to its optimal physical and mental performance.

Your brain literally minds your body and directs its functions, and the interrelationships of its glands, organs, tissues, and cells. It understands and anticipates the need of each of its members and tries to bring them in balance with each other, so that all parts or members may unite as one in a grand orchestral performance of body and spirit in perfect harmony. Therefore, every member and each cell thereof must receive the exact nutrients in the precise amounts required for their maximum output and their finest performance.

When your body needs potassium, your brain instructs you to eat a banana. When you need vitamin C, you become hungry for an orange. You have surely experienced the craving for various foods such as green salads, apples, broccoli, corn, oats, wheat, milk, and even chocolate. The brain never sends a message causing you to desire a pill containing vitamins and minerals, be they vitamin A, B, C, D, E, or K, or any other specific nutrients or combination of them. The brain does not care whether these nutrients are contained in a tablet or liquid; it was not programmed to function in that manner. The brain recognizes foods, by sight, aroma, touch, taste, and texture. Unfortunately, we may also crave sugar-containing candies and pastries, and as we all know, too much of these sweets are harmful to our body. Sugar (sucrose) is a substance that deceives the brain because it is rapidly converted into glucose by the body. Sugar is both the body's strength and its weakness. Glucose fuels both the brain and the body. When we consume too much of it and utilize too little, it builds up in our blood, causing damage to our organs and tissues. As you proceed through this book, you will learn how stevia helps to naturally reduce your cravings for sugar, and for sugar-containing sweets, and thus is so essential to health and vitality.

When you properly chew your food, or drink a beverage, you absorb some of its nutrients through the lining of your cheeks and from under your tongue. These nutrients are assimilated into your capillaries, carried to the carotid arteries in your neck, and transported directly to your brain, where they are thoroughly analyzed.

The brain manufactures and sends numerous neuropeptides throughout the body—to every gland, organ, tissue, and cell. Communication is constant between these special cells and the brain. While science does not yet fully comprehend all of the various functions of neuropeptides, at least one purpose, which is relevant to our discussion, appears evident. Some of these special warriors are agents of reconnaissance. They keep watch over the entire body, down to the smallest cell. Like guardian angels, they continuously report their findings to the brain.

When a problem is detected, the brain, in what to us is the subconscious mode, springs into action. It dispatches the necessary forces of the immune system to quell and eliminate the invasion of foreign materials, or sends the required nutrients and phytochemicals to restore your ill or undernourished cells. Your body, under the expert direction of its own maestro, has the ability to correct many of the disturbances and discords it encounters in its internal chorus. It can even rearrange or redesign its internal structure and connections according to your specific need. But to do so it must be appropriately and continuously fortified through proper and wise nourishment and use (exercise) of your entire being—body, mind, and spirit. Your body, if functioning correctly, is endowed with the ability to extract the precise nutrients from the foods you eat, in the correct amounts to nourish and maintain perfect cellular function. To facilitate this—that is, to keep your body functioning correctly—you need to nourish your body and brain with a variety of quality foods, specifically raw vegetables and fruits, which are rich in nutrients. You must also deny yourself the substances that will instill a dependency upon a specific chemical, or cause confusion in the processes of communication between the brain, mind, and spirit; thereby, doing long-range harm to your total being.

While they may be important for your condition, medicines are not something a normal brain will instinctively request. You may intellectually understand the benefits of a certain medicine, but unless it is an addictive substance that alters your body chemistry, your brain will not normally make you hunger for it. You have to *remember* to take them. You hunger, or have cravings, for foods: for apples, bananas, oranges, carrots, grapes, various berries, oats, wheat, and the like. Satisfy your hunger for *nourishing whole foods* and let your brain do the rest.

You may find that you will develop a desire for certain formulations of the wondrous food that is stevia. Some forms of stevia are wonderfully nutritious, while other forms do not contain the same nutritional value. However, stevia in each of its currently developed forms performs important functions for good within the human body.

WHOLE-LEAF STEVIA PRODUCTS

Dr. Pavvo Airola wrote the following wisdom in his book *How to Get Well* (Health Plus Publishers, 1988):

> Herbs have been used as healing agents since the beginning of time by every race upon the earth. Primitive people in every corner of this planet possessed remarkable knowledge of the medicinal value of certain roots, bark, seeds and plants that grew in their environment. . . . The records of Persian, Roman, Hebrew, Chinese and Egyptian medicine show that herbal medicine was in the highest regard and used extensively to cure practically every ill known to man.[1]

Information concerning the healing benefits of stevia and its sweetening characteristics is literally sweeping the world. Unfortunately most of the authors of these books and the writers of articles in various publications have not personally experienced these benefits. Their knowledge has often been gleaned from interviewing other people or from reading what other people have written. Generally, these journalists possess little firsthand knowledge. The result often leads to confusion and misunderstanding. All of the data in the remainder of this chapter is from what I have personally experienced; observed in my family, friends, and customers; had reported directly to me by mouth or pen; or read in published scientific research documents. That which I have studied in these documents, the assumptions made or conclusions reached by the scientists, I have seen either substantiated or refuted by human use.

Stevia Leaves

Green in color, quality stevia leaves are good for the body because they are highly nutritious. Stevia contains a number of important nutrients that are lacking in many of the foods we eat but that are vital to the ability of the various glands and organs of the body to function correctly, with precision and balance. Some of the nutrients thus far discovered in stevia are:

Aluminum	Niacin
Ascorbic acid	Phosphorus
Ash	Potassium
Austroinulin	Protein
Calcium	Rebaudioside
Beta-carotene	Riboflavin
Chromium	Selenium
Cobalt	Silicon
Dulcosides	Sodium
Fat	Stevioside
Fiber	Thiamin
Fluoride	Tin
Iron	Water
Magnesium	Zinc
Manganese	

During the 1970s various researchers found stevia leaves to contain eight diterpene glycosides, three nonsweet labdane diterpenes, two triterpenes, two sterols, a flavonoid (later identified as rutin), and unidentified tannins. They also discovered that stevia leaves contain an essential oil with fifty-three compounds, of which thirty-one were identified by 1980, including camphor and limonene. These oils include two alkanols, one aldehyde, one aromatic alcohol, twelve monoterpenes, and fifteen sesquiterpenes. At the time of this particular study (1977), twenty-two compounds remained unidentified, including four sesquiterpenes hydrocarbons, one sesquiterpene alcohol, and a ketone.[2] In 1983, A. Rajbhandari and M. F. Roberts, of London University, discovered that stevia leaves also contain the additional flavonoids of apignin, luteolin, kaempferol, quercitrin, and two forms of quercetin.[3,4,5] Other studies have demonstrated that steviol, the aglycone of stevioside, acts as a growth hormone (gibberellins) and stimulates the growth of certain vegetable-producing plants.[6] Although vitamin K has not yet been reported as having been found in stevia leaves, it is unquestionably present, because the vitamin is produced by the leaves of green plants in the process of photosynthesis. According to the USDA Human Nutrition Research Center on Aging at Tufts University in Boston, any green vegetation contains vitamin K.[7] Chlorophyll is also missing from the list, but it exists in all green plants and leaves, and is thus present in stevia. Since stevia is green plant material, it also contains carbohydrates in its leaves.

With so many vital nutrients, it is easy to see why stevia is good for the human body. Even though some of these nutrients may not be present in sufficient quantity to produce a therapeutic effect on their own, together they produce amazing results. The fact that premium-quality leaves can be about thirty times sweeter than sugar is merely a plus in stevia's favor. Perhaps, stevia was given its sweet taste to enhance the message of desirability, or "hunger," from brain to body.

Uses

Use stevia leaves to flavor and sweeten water, tea and other beverages, soups, sauces, and other foods. Freshen the mouth by placing a leaf on the tongue; the fresh and clean feeling can last for hours. Put one or more leaves between the cheek and gum as a tobacco substitute or simply for a long-lasting taste sensation. If you cannot find stevia leaves, simply remove a small amount of the contents of a tea bag and use in the same manner. While tobacco placed in the mouth causes disastrous results, stevia has never been shown, or even known, to cause harm of any kind. For maximum sensations of taste, it is best not to chew the whole leaves, which release bitter compounds from the veins that contain some of the constituents of healing. Unlike tobacco, if you happen to swallow some of the stevia material, so much the better. It's good for you. The "juice" should be swallowed, not expectorated.

Ground Stevia Leaves

Stevia leaves can be ground to what is referred to as "cut and sifted," which is the size used in tea bags, or to a fine spicelike powder. Both forms are excellent as a seasoning ingredient, with the fine powder being somewhat superior. Sprinkle the ground stevia on foods just as you would use other spices or seasonings. However, apply it sparingly; you can always add more. Ground stevia leaves not only add nutritional value to foods and beverages but also enhance their natural flavors while providing a gentle sweet taste. This product will quickly become a staple on your spice rack.

Uses

Sprinkle ground stevia leaves on vegetables or meats during cooking or while they are steaming hot. Heat enhances the release of the sweet flavor of stevia. Try ground stevia leaves in barbecue sauces, sweet and sour sauces, stews, soups, beans, chili, pizza, applesauce, and hot cereals. You will love them on baked or mashed potatoes, either alone or with other condiments. Add ground stevia leaves to bread or cookie dough, or sprinkle them on top of the dough prior to baking. Sprinkle them over green salads or add them to salad dressings. The uses for ground stevia leaves are as varied as your imagination.

Stevia Tea Bags

Stevia tea bags can be used to make a delicious and highly medicinal beverage. One tea bag can sweeten two to six cups of water or a lightly flavored beverage, depending upon the taste desired.

Because of the taste variance of other beverages, practice will quickly reveal the number of tea bags or stevia leaves required to obtain the degree of sweetness you prefer.

Uses

Use stevia tea bags to make stevia tea or to sweeten other beverages, hot or cold. Note that it takes much longer for the sweet glycosides in stevia to be released in a cold liquid than in a hot liquid. For cold beverages, it is always wise to first make stevia tea or stevia tea concentrate with steaming hot water. After three to five minutes, add ice to the hot liquid to speed the cooling process. When cool, add the tea or concentrate to other cold beverages as desired. Used in this manner, stevia functions as both a liquid nutritional supplement and a sweetener.

To prepare a mild concentrate, place one or more tea bags in a cup and cover with hot water. The more tea bags you use, the more water will be required. You can prepare a stronger concentrate by cooking the stevia at a very hot but not boiling temperature. Remove it from the heat and allow it to sit for three to five minutes or until cool enough to use. Store the concentrate in the refrigerator for future use. Stevia tea bags can also be placed directly in another beverage. Mothers report that frozen stevia tea makes a delicious and nutritious treat that is relished by children. Simply pour mild tea into a Popsicle mold and freeze it. Many mothers have reported that after a while they increased the nutritional value of the frozen treat by adding yerba maté tea to the stevia tea before freezing it. These two teas provide an extraordinary complement of the vitamins, minerals, and phytonutrients that are essential for children in a form that is delicious and easily assimilated into the body. Obviously, any other beverage can be added to the blend as well. Adjust the amount of stevia to achieve the sweetness most desired by the child. These stevia frozen treats will decrease your children's desire for other sweets while at the same time reducing their potential for cavities by improving their oral hygiene.

Note: When preparing herbal tea, you should always use steaming hot water. All foods, be they leaf material, roots, blossoms, fruits, or grains, are susceptible to the transport of bacteria. That is simply the natural course for foods grown in soil, water, and air. Unless the material is put through some sort of sterilizing process, some of these bacteria will remain on it. The sterilizing process itself may be more harmful to us than the bacteria. By preparing tea with hot water, you will eliminate sufficient bacteria so that the harm caused by those remaining becomes negligible. Once the tea is brewed, add ice or allow it to cool naturally, and then refrigerate it.

HEALING BENEFITS OF WHOLE-LEAF STEVIA PRODUCTS

Since modern man discovered stevia, his quest has been for the potential financial rewards of a safe, high-intensity sweetener. But the Guarani of Paraguay understood the real value of stevia. They learned about its incredible ability to heal the body, both internally and externally. The sweet taste of stevia is the least of its miraculous proprieties.

Appetite Control

Stevia, in its natural whole-leaf forms, helps to suppress the pangs of hunger, and to significantly reduce the craving for sugar-containing sweets of all kinds. You will still enjoy sweets but your intense craving for them will be lessened. Most people who use stevia daily tend to naturally reduce the amount of sweets they ingest. Self-control is no longer a problem, nor the lack thereof a detriment.

Blood Pressure

Some people have reported an apparent mild lowering of the blood pressure when using stevia daily. To my knowledge, this effect has not been documented medically or scientifically for whole-leaf stevia products, although it has been for stevia liquid concentrate.

Blood Sugar

A number of people have experienced a mild progression toward a balancing of their blood sugar when using stevia leaves, ground or whole, in their daily diet. This effect is more pronounced, however, with the use of stevia concentrate.

Colds and Flu

People who drink stevia tea or stevia-containing beverages on a daily basis report fewer incidences of colds and flu. This may be due to the inability of the viruses to digest the sweet glycosides, which naturally coat the throat upon swallowing the beverage. It may also be due to the natural zinc in stevia leaves. Medical research has demonstrated that zinc absorbed through the mouth and throat tends to kill viruses on contact. It could be a combination of both of these effects, or others not yet understood.

Dental Hygiene

People who use stevia daily in any of its forms have experienced a reduction in their number of dental caries and improved healing of bleeding gums. The bacteria that cause these conditions seem to love the sweet glycosides but cannot digest them and thus die. Therefore daily use of stevia results in a significant improvement in overall dental health and a freshening of the breath. (Bad breath is often caused by bacterial colonies on the back of the tongue.) Stevia should be the first line of defense against objectionable breath odors, cavities, and periodontal disease. There is significant scientific research that verifies the use of stevia for dental hygiene. (For a further discussion of this topic, see pages 84–85.)

Digestive Complaints

To quell an upset stomach, place one tea bag in a cup and add 8 to 12 ounces of steaming hot water. Allow the brew to steep until it has cooled enough to drink, about three to five minutes. Then drink the entire cup, preferably while still warm. In most situations, the result will be a rapid settling of the stomach. Stevia advocates have reported that this procedure has also been effective against food poisoning. As described above, the bacteria that cause upset stomach love stevia, but like humans, they cannot digest the sweet glycosides. Apparently, they continue to eat them until they starve to death. In the case of food poisoning, if drinking stevia tea does not bring rapid relief, consult a qualified physician.

Facial Wrinkles

After preparing stevia tea, place the wet tea bag over the eye so that it covers the wrinkles below and beside the eye. Allow the tea bag to remain in position for five minutes or longer. You will notice a smoothing of the wrinkles and a softening of the skin following this procedure.

Mental and Physical Stamina

Whole leaf stevia tends to increase physical stamina and mental acuity. You will notice a gentle increase in your physical and mental endurance, followed by no sudden letdown. Body builders have reported that dark whole-leaf concentrated liquid and stevia tablets are helpful in increasing strength and stamina.

Tobacco Addiction

Many people have reported that whole stevia leaves placed in the mouth reduced their desire to smoke cigarettes. Stevia, they say, was a significant aid in their effort to stop smoking. If stevia leaves were not available, some of these people opened a stevia tea bag and put a small amount of the dry tea leaves between their cheek and gum. However, even more people reported that they instead drank a hot cup of the yerba maté tea with stevia each time they felt the need for a cigarette, and achieved the same, if not better, results.

Weight Control

Because stevia contains no calories, helps to suppress the appetite, and reduces the desire for sweets, it can be very helpful in weight control. Stevia should be an essential part of the diet of anyone who wants to lose body fat or maintain current body weight. It must be noted, however, that eating stevia does not override the *habit* of eating sweets, nor the enjoyment thereof. However, most stevia users seem to feel satisfied with smaller portions of their favorite sweets. Use stevia products in place of all or most of the sugar or artificial sweeteners you use, either directly or in cooked or baked foods.

(For a discussion of aspartame and fat storage, see Chapter 6.)

SWEETENING CHARACTERISTICS OF WHOLE-LEAF STEVIA PRODUCTS

The sweetening capabilities of whole-leaf stevia products vary depending on the quality and cleanliness of the leaves. Quality is determined by the composition and arrangement of the various sweet constituents or glycosides in the leaves. The time of harvest is also critical to maintaining the sweet taste. If the plant blossoms, the sweetness of the leaves is reduced. Farmers cannot grow both premium quality leaves and produce seeds. They must make a choice. The leaves should be light green in color, not brown, and contain few, if any, stems. Commercially available leaves range in sweetness from about fifteen to thirty times that of sugar. The taste of some leaves is less than this because of foreign material, including dust, remaining on them. The sweetest leaves and whole-leaf products currently available on the commercial market are grown in South America. However, Chinese growers are making rapid progress in this area.

Use caution when buying whole stevia leaves. Examine them closely. Smell them. They should not smell like dirt. Some stevia leaves that have been sold in the United States have both smelled and tasted like dirt. Taste a leaf. Place it on your tongue. Do not bite or chew it; this will release the bitter (but healing) compounds

from the leaf veins. At first the sweet taste will be almost impercep-
tible, but as your saliva begins to soften the leaf, the sweet glycosides will be released. The delicate sweet flavor of a quality stevia
leaf will delight your tastebuds, and the sweetness will become
more and more profound over the next few minutes. When the
sweet taste is gone, you can swallow or expectorate the residue.

Stevia leaf residue has been shown to be an excellent source of
nutrients for livestock and plants, so don't just throw it away. Feed
it to your garden plants or your houseplants. Stevia literally is good
down to the last drop and to the last particle of leaf.

A final word of caution: As previously mentioned, stevia leaves
can carry a higher than desirable level of bacterial infestation. The
manner in which they were grown, harvested, cured, and processed
is critical. Know your source! Two or three leaves, or a little ground
stevia spice, will not carry enough bacteria to be problematic. However, when you use the equivalent of several leaves at a time, wisdom suggests making a tea with hot water, then using the tea for
sweetening other beverages. You can store the sweet tea in the refrigerator for several days of convenient use. Don't be overly concerned about a small amount of bacteria. Everything natural, including
our bodies, always carries bacteria, and our bodies are designed to
handle these normal amounts of bacteria.

This does propose somewhat of a dilemma. If stevia kills harmful bacteria, how can bacteria live on the surface of the leaves?
While this has not yet been addressed by scientific research, there
is an apparent and simple answer. You will remember that it is the
sweet stevioside and rebaudioside glycosides, when ingested, that
kill bacteria by starvation. These glycosides are encapsulated
within the cellular structure of the leaves and are released only
when the leaves are soaked in water or another liquid. Therefore,
only a fairly concentrated aqueous solution of stevia or pure stevioside or rebaudioside will kill bacteria. When stevia leaves or tea bag
material is held in the mouth for several minutes, the saliva acts as
the aqueous solution, causing the release of the sweet glycosides.

Stevia is truly a gift coming from the wisdom of the ancients. It
will add new dimensions of natural healing to anyone willing to ex-

perience it in its various forms. The more I have learned of and experienced the miracle of stevia, the more determined I have become to make it available to North Americans. The Guarani people, however, were most excited about the internal and topical healing properties of stevia concentrate. I was soon to understand their enthusiasm.

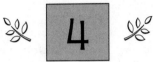

Healing Balm of the Guarani: Stevia Concentrate

"Nothing is obvious to the uninformed." —Anonymous

Because of the numerous uses and wonderful medicinal qualities of water-based stevia concentrate, and the incredible results obtained from its use, I am devoting this chapter to this magnificent liquid stevia. I will relate personal experiences from my life, from the lives of members of my family, and from grateful consumers.

When the Guarani developed this form of stevia, they created a blessing for the entire world. I had seen it used and was told about its miraculous healing benefits during my first trip to Paraguay. I didn't believe the stories. However, I was willing to try it as a sweetener and so brought a few bottles with me when I returned to Arizona.

THE PERFECT TRIAL

My first experience with the healing power of stevia concentrate came in 1983. I had taken my family to an all-you-can-eat restaurant. It was located at the intersection of two main traffic arteries in Scottsdale, Arizona. As we were about to enter the building, I noticed a car stalled in the middle of the intersection. The lone occupant was a woman. With cars whizzing past her in every direction, she was obviously frightened and didn't know what to do. She needed help.

Even though my sons were then quite young, I said, "Come on, boys, let's push her out of the intersection." I took off with my three sons right behind me. With the traffic stopped at the light, I leaped off the curb into the street at a dead run. Since my attention was focused on the woman and the traffic, I didn't notice the loose gravel in the road. My feet went out from under me and I fell hard, face forward, sliding on the gravel and asphalt pavement, made burning hot by the scorching summer sun. I put out my hands to break the fall and my right hand, at the base of the thumb, was badly torn and embedded with tiny gravel fragments. Attention now became focused on Dad, who was a bloody mess. By the time my boys helped me up and were trying to get me out of the street, traffic had again started toward us. No one slowed down. However, someone in a car was pushing the lady in distress to safety.

Everyone thought we should cancel our dinner and go to the emergency room of the nearby hospital. Everyone except me. I didn't want to spoil the family's afternoon out. Besides, everyone was famished. Can you imagine five hungry children waiting in a hospital emergency room? The trauma of that would have been far worse on the family than my injury was to me. I said that I would go to the emergency room following dinner, after taking the family home. I brushed myself off with my left hand, and with the help of my sons, went into the rest room of the restaurant. I washed the wound, rinsed the blood from my hand and arm, and picked out the gravel particles as best I could. After the bleeding had stopped and my hand was wrapped in a clean handkerchief, we enjoyed our meal.

Upon arriving home, I examined the wound more closely, dug out the remaining gravel, and washed the hand thoroughly. Remembering what I had been told about stevia concentrate in Paraguay, I decided that this was the perfect time to put it to the test. I poured the liquid concentrate into the open wound.

I was not prepared for what happened. My Paraguayan mentors had warned that it would sting a little. They were wrong. It really hurt! I grabbed my stevia-covered hand and moaned aloud, "Oh, why did I ever do this?" It was just like pouring iodine into an open cut—except that in about forty-five seconds the pain went away. There was no pain. There was no discomfort. It was as if there were no wound. I bandaged my hand and forgot about it for the rest of the evening. The healing was incredibly rapid, and the wound left no scar. I was amazed. And now—the *rest* of the story.

STEVIA CONCENTRATE PRODUCTS

Since I first brought stevia concentrate to America, many companies, recognizing either its healing properties or profit potential, have created similar products, which they sell in health food stores or through network marketing programs. Some of these products are good while some are not. In my opinion, the product should be water-based, not prepared with alcohol. A properly made product will have wonderful healing effects.

Currently, stevia concentrate is available in two primary forms: whole-leaf stevia concentrate and whole-leaf stevia concentrate tablets.

Whole-Leaf Stevia Concentrate

To make concentrate, whole-leave stevia is cooked, through a special procedure, until it is highly concentrated in a base of pure water. Stevia concentrate is dark in color and looks somewhat like molasses. To be effective, it must have a relatively thick consistency. If thin like water, it will not be as effective. Stevia concentrate has the same benefits as whole-leaf stevia discussed in Chapter 3, but because it is highly concentrated, the *results are much more profound.* Also, stevia in this form has many additional benefits not obtained from the leaves themselves.

Stevia concentrate is a food. It tastes like licorice but has numerous medicinal uses. It is both wise and convenient to keep stevia concentrate in the bathroom medicine cabinet, in your travel kit, and in the kitchen. Because harmful bacteria cannot survive in the concentrate, it does not require refrigeration after opening. It will last for years without spoiling or losing its effectiveness. You may discover, as have so many others, that after gaining some experience with this remarkable healing liquid, you will come to consider it your first choice for many medical emergencies. Those experienced in its use suggest that no home should be without at least two bottles at all times. As you read about the incredible uses for this product, you will understand the enthusiasm many people share with the Guarani natives of Paraguay.

Uses

A few drops of stevia concentrate will sweeten nearly any beverage. Coffee, however, may require a little more than other drinks. According to Rogelio Valdez Benegas, Ph.D., a recently retired biochemist with the College of Chemistry, University of Asunción, Paraguay, this is because the sweet compounds in stevia, as arranged in the whole leaf or liquid concentrate, do not bind well with caffeine, thus requiring additional drops to overcome coffee's bitterness. If a few more drops are required to sweeten your coffee, just consider them to be bringing you extra health benefits.

Stevia concentrate is especially useful in acidic beverages such as lemonade, as it remains effective within the pH range of 3 to 9. (The pH scale measures acidity and alkalinity.) It is also an excellent addition to aloe vera concentrate and beverages. One drop in a one- or two-ounce "shot" of pure aloe juice usually nullifies the unpleasant taste. Two drops make the juice palatable. A blend of these two herbs—aloe and stevia—is highly beneficial to the human body, both internally and topically.

Stevia concentrate also works well in drinks made from either powdered or liquid concentrate. It can be used to sweeten hot and cold breakfast cereals by adding a few drops to the milk. The only downside to using stevia concentrate is that it adds a dark color and a slight licoricelike flavor to beverages and foods. The specific color and flavor vary according to the ratio of the concentrate to the beverage or food. However, mothers often suggest serving children milk nutritionally fortified and sweetened with several drops of stevia concentrate. They say it looks similar to chocolate milk and tastes even better.

For a health-promoting, power-packed, but delicious beverage, place two or three tea bags of yerba maté in a tall cup or glass and add hot milk or soymilk. Stir in stevia concentrate to taste and allow the beverage to steep for several minutes. When removing the tea bags, squeeze them gently against the side of the cup with a spoon to release the remaining flavor and nutrients. Serve the drink hot or cold.

Whole-Leaf Stevia Concentrate Tablets

Whole-leaf stevia concentrate tablets are dark in color and a little thicker than aspirin tablets. They are produced by concentrating liquid concentrate even more and then eliminating the water. The dry stevia nutrients are pressed together with oat bran and retain a strong licorice flavor, which overpowers any sweet taste. They are a convenient-to-carry form of highly concentrated stevia but have little use as a sweetener. (Each tablet equals about thirty drops of stevia concentrate.) They should be swallowed with water as needed.

Uses

The primary use for stevia concentrate tablets is to nourish the pancreas and to balance pancreatic activity. They dissolve rapidly and, like the liquid, will assist the body in normalizing blood sugar. This, of course, will help to increase energy when the blood sugar is low. Many people prefer to carry a few tablets around with them rather than a bottle of liquid. The benefits within the body are similar to those provided by the liquid. Athletes who engage in strenuous activity, diabetics, hypoglycemics, and anyone who is prone to experiencing a sudden drop or rise in blood glucose find them easy to carry, allowing them to be readily available when needed either for increased energy or for balancing blood sugar.

HEALING BENEFITS OF STEVIA CONCENTRATE

The healing benefits of stevia concentrate include those for whole-leaf stevia described in Chapter 3. The effects, however, are more profound. Stevia concentrate also has a number of additional benefits.

Appetite Control

Because of its concentration, whole-leaf stevia concentrate appears to be the most effective form of stevia for appetite suppression. People have reported that taking stevia drops fifteen to twenty minutes before a meal decreases their hunger sensations, helping them to eat less.

A most interesting corollary to this comes from Tobin Watkinson, D.C., of San Diego, California. Following a visit to my office a few years ago, to learn more about stevia, he incorporated it into his practice of nutrition and nutritional research in his Scripps medical clinic. After several months he called me to report the experiences of his patients. They were eating less and losing weight. As he researched the phenomenon, he developed a very plausible theory. With excitement in his voice, he said, "I think that stevia resets the pathway between the stomach and the hypothalamus [the gland that regulates hunger and thirst, among other things]." Realizing that I might not understand his statement or his enthusiasm, he clarified his conclusion: "Jim, when we eat and are satiated, a signal is transmitted between the stomach and the hypothalamus, enabling the brain to tell us we have eaten enough. The desire to eat is shut off. We think that many people are obese because this signal is somehow interrupted. There is a blockage somewhere in the system. Without this signal, people just keep on eating long after they are satiated. They gain weight, sometimes becoming enormously obese, simply because they don't know they have eaten enough. We think that the stevia concentrate is somehow resetting this mechanism."

He wanted me to engage a university research center to prove his theory. Unfortunately, had I done so, and the theory was proven correct, stevia concentrate would have been classified as a medicine rather than a nutritional supplement. As a medicine, the FDA would remove it from the market as an unapproved drug. The fact that it was effective and might improve the health and perhaps even extend the lives of hundreds of thousands, or even millions, of people at a very low cost would not matter. It would be required to go through their approval process, costing hundreds of millions of dollars and years of delay.

Because stevia concentrate is a natural product, it cannot be patented. However, if a drug were made from stevia or synthesized, the drug could be patented, but the natural product could continue to be sold, reducing the potential market for the approved medicine. The FDA might then go along with the pharmaceutical company and remove the natural stevia from the market thereby protecting the profits of the drug manufacturer. There is no way to win this battle. It is a true catch-22, and the people who suffer from the numerous maladies, conditions, and diseases that stevia could help are the losers.

Bleeding Gums

In other countries, stevia is added to commercial toothpastes and mouthwashes, but in the United States, the FDA does not allow this. However, many people use the concentrate (probably the most effective form for oral hygiene) as a mouthwash and also add two or three drops to their regular toothpaste when brushing their teeth. (Stevia extract powder can also be added to toothpaste; see Chapter 5.) The dark stevia concentrate will discolor your toothbrush, but that's a small price to pay for improved oral hygiene. Numerous people (including myself) report that when adding ten to twelve drops to a mouthful of water and swishing vigorously, on a regular basis, their gums stop bleeding. You can just swish and swallow, or if you prefer, you can expectorate. You will also be left with a clean, refreshing taste and feeling in your mouth.

Research has demonstrated that stevia significantly reduces plaque, which is a bacterial infestation. Recent research has also indicated that there may be a link between heart attacks and bacterial-caused gum disease resulting in inflammation of the blood vessels. Stevia's ability to kill oral bacteria might prove beneficial with this medical condition as well.

Blood Pressure

Scientific research has indicated that stevia in an "aqueous solution"—that is, water-based stevia concentrate—appeared to lower high blood pressure but seemingly had no effect on normal blood pressure. While many scientists and the FDA are not willing to accept this apparent benefit, it has been borne out repeatedly by consumers. Almost invariably people who add stevia to their daily diet *and* use the dark stevia concentrate each day experience a reduction in high blood pressure.

One story will suffice: A man called me from Texas. He was really excited about what had happened to him the day before. He said he had hypertension and had felt strange, but being a salesman and working on commission, he had to continue to make his normal calls. By afternoon the feeling had gotten much worse. He really felt weird and his head had begun pounding. He finally realized that he'd better get to his doctor. When he got there, they rushed him into an examining room, had him lie on the table, and took his blood pressure. After examining him, the doctor said his blood pressure was so high that he could have died at any minute. The doctor had him stay on the table for a while. When he returned to the examining room, he again took the man's blood pressure and said it was still dangerously high. He gave the man a prescription and took him out to the waiting room. He told the man to sit there in an easy chair for a while and then, when he felt able, to walk carefully and slowly to his car, and to go home and lie down immediately. He again cautioned the man, saying that his blood pressure had been so high that any rapid movement or excitement could have killed him. He said that it was still dangerously high.

When the man got to his car, he remembered that there was a bottle of stevia concentrate in the glove compartment. Recalling an article he had read about stevia lowering high blood pressure, he decided to try it and see if it would help. He swallowed two tablespoonfuls and then just sat in his car for thirty minutes. Within a few minutes he began to feel better. Everything was calming down. At the end of the half-hour, he returned to his doctor's office and asked the doctor to check his blood pressure again. He told him that he felt much better and that he thought it must have gone down. After checking it, the doctor looked at him with a very puzzled expression, and said, "I don't understand it but your blood pressure is normal." The man then told him what he had done. The doctor said that he'd never seen anything like it in all of his practice. He also told him to keep using the stevia. "Believe me," the man said to me, "I intend to. I'm going to keep it with me all the time."

This account is very unusual and may not be a typical reaction. We are all different. While these and dozens of similar experiences have convinced me of the value of stevia concentrate for lowering high blood pressure, its use should not replace competent medical advice and practice. It is, however, well worth a try. It is completely safe, with no harmful side effects.

In *The Stevia Cookbook,* Ray Sahelian, M.D., and Donna Gates report the following:

> In 1991, Dr. M. S. Melis, from the Department of Biology at the University of São Paulo in Brazil, did a study to determine the effects of stevioside on blood pressure. After giving a one-time high-dose injection of stevioside to a group of laboratory rats, he found that they experienced a reduction in blood pressure as well as an increased elimination of sodium (Melis 1991). A slight diuretic effect also occurred. The effect was even stronger when stevia was combined with verapamil, a medicine commonly prescribed for lowering blood pressure.
>
> In a similar study in 1995, Dr. Melis administered oral doses of stevia to lab rats for up to sixty days. After twenty days, there were no changes in the stevia-treated rats compared to those who did not receive the extract. However, after both forty and sixty days of administering the stevia, the rats showed a reduction in blood pressure, a diuretic effect, and an increase in sodium loss. The amount of blood going to the kidneys was also increased (Melis).
>
> One small study in Brazil involved eighteen average, healthy human volunteers between the ages of twenty and forty years. After the test subjects were given tea prepared with stevia leaves for thirty days, a ten percent lowering of blood pressure occurred (Boeck).[1]

Blood Sugar

Stevia concentrate is far and away the most effective form of stevia for helping to restore correct blood sugar balance. Most people who have tried this product report a rapid correction of blood glucose imbalance. For people with hypoglycemia, pancreatic response is usually evident within several minutes. Diabetics often report a positive response within a few days. Obviously, if people do not have a dramatically positive response, they do not call with any accolades. We, therefore, do not know what percent of those who try stevia have good results. Let a few stories suffice.

Diabetes

A man called from the Midwest. He had heard about stevia concentrate and wanted information and instructions regarding its use. He said that his blood sugar was 240 and nothing was helping to lower it. I explained that I was neither a doctor nor a scientist, and could only repeat what others had reported, without knowledge as to the truthfulness of their claims. Further, I had no way of knowing, nor could it be implied, that he would have results similar to those reported by these individuals. He understood. He asked how many drops he should use and how often each day. I replied that I could not give that information because it would be construed as prescribing a medication. Now he was really frustrated and began to become angry.

With some degree of trepidation, I suggested that I could tell him how a friend had explained how he was using the concentrate, with apparent success. This friend had reported that he squeezed a lemon into a tall glass, added thirty drops of stevia concentrate, stirred, and then filled the glass with cold water and drank it all. He followed this procedure three times each day, immediately after his meals. The man said, "Great! I'll try that." I cautioned him that he should monitor his blood glucose levels often. If his count dropped too rapidly, he might want to reduce the number of stevia drops. I also suggested that he inform his physician of the experiment.

About a week later I got another phone call from the man. He said that the first day he drank the thirty drops with each of his three meals. The following morning his blood sugar level had dropped so much that he reduced the stevia to twenty drops. With the rapid reduction continuing, he went to ten drops on the third day. He gleefully shouted, "And on the fourth day my blood sugar was normal!" He had discovered that for him, ten drops with each meal maintained a normal glucose level.

The following day I got a phone call from a lady in New Jersey. She wanted to relate her mother's experience. Her mother's blood sugar level was 300 and she had told her to use ten to twelve drops of stevia concentrate three times each day. But since the mother knew nothing about stevia, she wisely called her medical doctor and got an appointment for the following afternoon to discuss whether or not she should continue to use it. By the time she saw the doctor, she had taken the suggested number of drops about five times.

She showed her physician the bottle of stevia concentrate. After reading the label, he admitted that he was not familiar with the herb. When he checked her blood sugar and found it normal, however, he told her to continue taking the stevia every day. He suggested that if her blood sugar remained normal, she should reduce the number of drops each day until her blood glucose began to rise again. This way she could determine the fewest drops required for her blood sugar to remain normal. Through this experiment the woman determined that she required only about five to ten drops each day. Since, to my knowledege, there has never been a report of anyone having an adverse experience from using stevia, as much as desired can be used to flavor or sweeten foods. The pancreatic effect is merely a wonderful side benefit of the daily use of stevia.

The greatest fear that I have ever experienced with diabetics experimenting with stevia concentrate was in the early years, when the product was marketed and labeled solely for use in skin care. People would read articles about stevia and hear stories related by other diabetics or friends and decide to try stevia concentrate. After a few days of use they would call and with great excitement claim that their blood sugar had dropped so much that they had either reduced or discontinued their physician-prescribed insulin. The reply I would always give them was that neither they nor I were doctors, and they must *not* stop taking their insulin, nor reduce the amount, without their physician's knowledge and instructions. I would then instruct them to call their doctor, get an immediate, emergency appointment, and follow the physician's instructions.

Invariably, these people would call back a few days later and say that the doctor had either reduced or taken them off their insulin with instructions to continue with the stevia concentrate. The most soul satisfying of all of these experiences was the woman who had heard about stevia from a friend who had been encouraging her to try it. Her doctor had just told her that her leg needed to be amputated due to her diabetes. She was desperate and willing to try anything. I told her that there was no way to know if stevia concentrate would help her condition but that it would not hurt her if she wanted to try it.

How much stevia concentrate she used I do not know. Her friend suggested that she swallow the stevia by the teaspoonful, plus add it to everything she ate. When she called me a few weeks later, I could hardly understand her through the sobs and tears. The doctor had taken her off insulin and her leg had improved so much that amputation was no longer required. For the first time in years she could walk, albeit with a walker. Others have related similar experiences.

A few weeks ago, a friend and neighbor who is a diabetic and must take insulin daily suffered a severe and rapid onset of low blood sugar while teaching a religious class I was attending. He could no longer think clearly and became dizzy. He asked, "Does anyone have a candy bar?" A class member, apparently with the same condition, opened his briefcase and passed up a bar of candy, which my friend quickly devoured. One bar was not enough, however, and he asked for a second bar, which he ate. We waited and within a few minutes he was able to continue. We all suggested that he go home and take care of himself. We knew that his blood sugar would soon rise, requiring an injection of insulin. He insisted on completing the lesson, which was about Jesus telling the parable of the Good Samaritan bandaging the wounds of and caring for the man he found on the side of the road who had been attacked by thieves (Luke 10: 25–37).

On several previous occasions I had hinted to my friend that stevia might be beneficial to him. He had rejected the idea and thrown away the stevia concentrate that I had given him. Following church, I "girded up my loins" and telephoned him. I said: "In class today you taught us that a true friend and neighbor will bind up the wounds of the one who is suffering. You quoted the words of Jesus, saying, 'Go thou and do likewise.' I am your neighbor and your friend. I am coming over to bind up your wounds."

As we visited, I told him that after witnessing his distress, I decided it was time I shared with him what I knew to be true. He became very interested and we discussed the possible benefits of stevia for more than an hour. He said, "I want to try it." I gave him a bottle of concentrate and several other forms of stevia. I told him to be sure to go to his physician, tell him what he was doing, and follow the doctor's medical advice. A few days later he called to report that the stevia had been a significant help. He now required less insulin to lower his blood sugar.

Miracles? Tall tales? You must judge for yourself. I never kept any official records of these stories, nor have I ever written about them, for fear of reprisal by the FDA or the AMA. I did synopsize them in my telephone notes, however, and have had them permanently recorded in my brain, because I never cease to be amazed at the incredible benefits people experience from what I believe to be a wonderful gift from God.

Physicians often call me to learn about stevia and the other herbs of Paraguay. These medical doctors thank me for bringing these herbs to the United States and for the healing that they have observed in their patients or even in themselves. They are fascinated by what they have seen. When I express my hope that they tell their other patients about the herbs, their response is nearly always the same: "I can't. I dare not tell anyone. Your herbs are not approved as sound medical practice. The AMA would take away my membership." How sad.

Fortunately, naturopathic physicians can suggest stevia without fear of retribution from the AMA. Today, doctors who practice holistic medicine in many different countries, enthusiastically recommend stevia for blood sugar problems, as well as for a host of other conditions. One of the first of these physicians, who was introduced to stevia in 1994 and tested it on himself before recommending it to patients, was Julian Whitaker, M.D., founder of the Whitaker Wellness Institute in Newport Beach, California. In his highly informative book *Reversing Diabetes,* he writes:

> [Stevia] comes in several forms. The unrefined, dark extract is probably the healthiest way to go. It has even been shown in studies to improve blood sugar control. . . . You can use as much of this unique sweetener as you would like. It will not raise your blood sugar levels, and, if you use the unrefined extract, may actually lower them.[2]

While stevia is a food, if diabetics want to experience favorable results, they should ingest it regularly and frequently as if it were a medicine. This will enable the nutrients in stevia to act upon their body in a continuous manner, which is crucial to the healing process.

Hypoglycemia

People with low blood sugar seem to respond to stevia concentrate within several minutes. This was dramatically proven by my own daughter Erin. She and an older brother, Michael, were born with a condition known as phenylketonuria (PKU). In PKU, the liver does not produce the enzymes required to convert phenylalanine (one of the three chemicals used to formulate aspartame) into other chemicals necessary for the body. While the brain requires a small amount of phenylalanine for proper development, it will suffer permanent and irreversible brain damage from too much. Because of this, most children with PKU became permanently mentally retarded.

Children with PKU cannot eat protein because of its phenylalanine content. Their diet must be severely restricted, and at the time my children were young they had to ingest a synthetic powdered food blended with water into a milklike substance. When my children were infants, and as they grew up, only one such product was available. It was the most horrible-tasting stuff imaginable. If the infant or young child of friends who were visiting with us would pick up one of their bottles and take a swallow, the child would immediately gag and throw up.

Both Michael and Erin also had severe hypoglycemia. Erin's low blood sugar was even worse than her brother's. When she was five to six years old, I was learning about stevia and had begun importing and selling it in teas and in its dark liquid concentrate form. Protein was important for her severe hypoglycemic condition but would be disastrous to her brain because of the PKU. She would pass out almost daily and often go into convulsions. Nothing we tried prevented these episodes. Treatment for either medical condition made the other one worse. We were constantly rushing her to the emergency room but to no avail. The doctors there never knew what to do, and when we would try to explain the condition and what needed to be done, the arrogant but ignorant response was, "I'm the doctor here and she is now my patient." In those days most doctors knew nothing about PKU. Some had received a little training, but few understood the condition. Those were terrible and frightening times.

Upon the advice of our pediatrician, my wife took Michael and Erin to the medical research clinics at several different universities. Finally, one group of doctors *theorized* that Erin's severe low blood sugar was caused by microscopic tumors in her pancreas. They wanted to operate immediately. They wanted to open her up and cut slices from her pancreas. Each slice would be examined under a microscope until the suspected tumors were found. This procedure would continue, if necessary, until the entire pancreas was removed. Obviously, Erin would be on the operating table, at risk for her life, for hours. The doctors wanted to perform the same procedure on Michael. Although he had experienced significant improvement in recent months, he, too, had passed out from time to time and had also experienced grand mal seizures.

When my wife called and explained what the doctors wanted to do, I refused to allow the surgery. I told her to get the children out of that hospital and to come home. She called back, however, and said the doctors had told her that if I did not let them operate, the next episode could destroy Erin's brain. My daughter would be a vegetable—and it would be *my fault*. I told her to get Erin and

Michael out of that hospital anyway, with or without the approval of the doctors. They caught the next plane home.

In today's world some ill-advised judge might order me arrested and imprisoned for child abuse for not allowing the medical procedure determined appropriate by the doctors. I had served as a consultant to research physicians for several years and I felt strongly that their true interest was not the well-being or even the life of my daughter and son. She and Michael were the only two people in the world (known at that time) with the specific variant of PKU and hypoglycemia that they exhibited. Even more perplexing—and interesting—to the doctors was that their reactions differed from each other. Even though both had experienced repeated high levels of phenylalanine, it appeared that neither had suffered brain damage. Their cases were unique—and medically fascinating. I was convinced that these doctors just wanted to experiment and publish their findings. Their primary interest was personal fame and glory. Perhaps, however, their desires were due to the medical ignorance of the times.

Because of what I was learning at the time, I wanted to give Erin stevia concentrate to try to help her. All of the doctors had refused to allow me to give an unknown substance to *their* patient. I discussed the problem with a medical doctor who was also a close friend. He said, "Jim, what do you care what those doctors think? She is your daughter. You are responsible for her. If you think stevia might help her, try it. What have you got to lose?" With his encouragement I began to add six drops of stevia concentrate to the horrible-tasting concoction she had to drink daily for her PKU condition.

Erin had always hated the taste of the PKU stuff and it took hours to coax, plead, demand, and finally force her to drink it. It was a battle of the wills that she often won. Rarely could we get her to drink it all. When she was an infant, she gagged and vomited every time she tasted the liquid from her bottle, so I would have to hold her still while my wife inserted a tube through her nose and into her stomach. We would then force-feed the foul-tasting beverage directly into her stomach with a syringe, bypassing her taste sensations and gag reflexes. This procedure was repeated for every feeding during her infancy. It was hell for all three of us.

We had tried flavoring the PKU concoction with everything we could think of to diminish its bad taste but nothing helped. But the first time I prepared the drink with stevia concentrate, Erin took a sip through a straw, looked up at me, and said, "Gee, Dad, this isn't bad. What did you put in it this time?" I continued to add six drops of stevia concentrate to the drink every day. Both Erin and Michael drank the PKU beverage until they were about twelve or thirteen years old. The prevailing medical opinion was that by that age, the brain is developed and no longer in danger of significant damage. To the best of my knowledge, Erin did not experience a convulsion, nor pass out from low blood sugar from the day she began drinking the beverage with the added stevia concentrate. And those doctors had insisted that her pancreas needed to be removed or she would become a vegetable.

Later I learned that there had been a 25 percent chance that Erin and Michael would have died on the operating table and a 25 percent chance that they would have died following the surgery. At that time, life without a pancreas was miserable for a child, and such a child had a life expectancy that was very, very short, perhaps only two years. I still believe that these doctors were willing to sacrifice my daughter and son for their own experiments and the knowledge that they might have gained and the fame they had hoped to obtain.

At the time I first added the stevia concentrate to the PKU beverage, Erin was six. She is now twenty-five years old and a graduate of the University of Utah, with plans to continue on to graduate school. We thank God for His loving kindness. He gave us Erin and Michael, and then stevia and the wisdom to use it.

While Erin's brother Michael was willing to put up with the foul taste of the medicinal beverage, he loved the taste of yerba maté tea sweetened with stevia and drank large amounts every day. He is a graduate, with honors, of Brigham Young University, and is currently working toward his doctorate degree at Kansas State University. Only his dissertation remains to be completed. He plans to be a professor of history, specializing in military history, writing books and perhaps teaching in a university setting or serving as an advisor to the government on the history of war.

While the experience of Erin and Michael is not typical, the incidence of low blood sugar among the general population of the United States and Europe is incredibly high. In her excellent book *Living Food for Health,* Dr. Gillian McKeith, of London, England, an enthusiastic advocate of stevia, writes:

> Many patients I see are prone to hypoglycaemia and diabetes, the two major forms of blood sugar disorders which can deservedly be called modern day plagues. In fact, from my own clinical practice, I have found that one out of every two patients has either displayed hypoglycaemic symptoms at some time in the past, or has been clearly diagnosed with hypoglycaemia. The "over-sugarisation" (to coin my own term) of the general population has resulted in a situation whereby at least 50 per cent are at risk of hypoglycaemia. Hypoglycaemia can cause mood swings, irritability, depression, fatigue, drowsiness, tremors, headaches, dizziness, panic attacks, indigestion, cold sweats, even alcoholism and fainting. The brain needs adequate blood sugar to work properly; but if blood sugar levels wildly fluctuate, it can lead to such a litany of adverse symptoms.[3]

To maintain a healthy blood sugar balance, Dr. McKeith recommends the daily ingestion of stevia, which she considers to be a *superfood.* If 50 percent of our population has a blood sugar imbalance, is it possible this may be an underlying cause of, or at least a contributing factor to, the numerous symptoms being exhibited by millions of people today? Could wildly fluctuating blood glucose levels be the underlying cause of lethargy in children, or their inability to concentrate or to sit still, or the irritability that so many exhibit at school and home? When I was young, and before the American food supply was so overly sweetened with sugar, these behavior problems were virtually nonexistent. In school, behavior problems simply were not tolerated.

Just think about what schoolchildren today eat and what they do between the sugar-filled snacks that substitute as meals. For breakfast they have presweetened cereal or a sweet pastry—if they eat at all. Sugar is often the main ingredient in these cereals. They load up on sugar and arrive at school bursting with energy, but are expected to sit quietly and use their minds instead of their bodies. Then their blood sugar drops and they are lethargic and unable to think clearly let alone concentrate. For lunch they again stock up on sugar-laden junk foods and the process repeats itself. At home they sit and watch television or play video games until it's time for bed. They get little, if any, exercise.

All day long kids crave sugar-filled foods and carbohydrates—a sure indication of low blood sugar. Immediately after eating these sugary foods, their blood glucose soars and then falls through the floor. Dr. McKeith suggests that stevia could provide a significant but natural change in their eating habits and an attendant reduction in these dangerously fluctuating blood sugar episodes. She writes:

> In my own practice, I use stevia on those patients with a real sweet tooth—the type of person who is absolutely addicted to anything with sugar. In almost every case, the patient reports either a substantial reduction in cravings, or in some cases, a complete eradication of the sweet cravings. Several patients pointed out that they were able to curb other cravings as well. For example, one man who felt he needed pasta every day, suddenly didn't feel the need for it so desperately once on the stevia. He felt more balanced. When the blood sugar levels are regulated, our cravings for certain types of foods should regulate too.[4]

This is one more example of how the quality of the food you eat is critical to your health now—and perhaps even more importantly, to the quality of your life in the years to come.

Burns

I first heard of stevia concentrate being used to heal burns from the Guarani people in Paraguay. However, despite having used it often on cuts and abrasions, I have never had the opportunity to try it myself on a severe burn. So this story comes from a naturopathic physician, Dr. Louise Gutowski, of Scottsdale, Arizona. Dr. Gutowski has incorporated several Paraguayan herbal products into her practice. Because she has found them to be helpful, she simply recommends the ones she feels are appropriate for the particular symptoms. She called me to relate this story, then came to my office to retell the experience—twice.

A patient arrived at Dr. Gutowski's office with a serious burn. His car had overheated, and when he removed the radiator cap, the boiling water had spewed up and onto his arm. The arm was bright red, but the burn under where his metal watch had been was severe and the skin was badly blistered. After examining the damage to his flesh, the doctor poured stevia concentrate over the area. She said he immediately yelled and wrenched in pain. She had forgotten the stinging that lasts for a few seconds, and in this case, minutes, after applying the concentrate.

Dr. Gutowski apologized to the patient for causing him such discomfort. She told him she was confident the stevia concentrate would both prevent an infection and speed up the healing process. She gave him a bottle of the concentrate and told him to wait two or three days until the flesh was not so raw and the concentrate wouldn't sting, and then to begin applying it.

The next afternoon the patient telephoned her. He said, "I want to come and see you right now. I have to show you my arm." She was nervous over his call and afraid that perhaps the burn had gotten worse. When he arrived, he displayed an arm with no blisters or evidence of severe burns. It was just pink. As she looked at the arm, so badly burned just twenty-four hours earlier, she asked, "What did you do?" With a big grin on his face, he replied, "Well, after I got home, I got to thinking about what you said about the stevia healing my burn. Since I knew it would really hurt for a few minutes, I figured I could stand it, especially if it would heal faster. So I put some on the burn and then just kept putting more on all day. As soon as I got up this morning, I started again. And now it's well! That stuff is incredible!" Needless to say, Dr. Gutowski continues to recommend stevia concentrate to her patients. Other people have related similar stories of how stevia concentrate healed severe burns.

Cuts and Abrasions

If you have a cut or wound, first remove all the dirt and foreign particles from it. Then add sufficient drops of stevia concentrate to fill the opening and run over onto the skin. Be aware that this is going to sting, much like iodine would. However, after about forty-five seconds the stinging sensation will stop and there will be a significant reduction in the normal pain and discomfort of the wound. Some people report that they never feel pain again from the cut. Stevia concentrate causes a stinging sensation only when applied to raw, open flesh. A chiropractor reported that he severely cut the base of his thumb on the lid of a can of food that he was opening for lunch. He applied the stevia concentrate, bandaged the wound, and ate lunch. He called to report the incident because he was so astounded that, following lunch, he could perform the required manipulation on his patients and feel no pain or discomfort.

Wisdom suggests that you allow the stevia concentrate to dry within and over the cut. It will form a protective seal. When it wears or washes away, apply more concentrate. You will be amazed at how fast the cut will heal. You will notice that the cut is healing from the inside—that is, from the deepest point of the cut flesh—outward toward the skin. Doctors have called to report that they could almost see the flesh knitting itself back together. Interestingly, no scab will form, and no scar will remain. After experiencing the rapid healing and the lessening of long-term pain, even children prefer to tolerate the initial short-term discomfort.

As I have already described, my use of stevia for cuts and wounds began in 1983. I learned of the incredible sterilizing and healing effects of stevia concentrate from the natives of Paraguay. Since that time, I have used nothing but stevia concentrate for the numerous cuts and tearings of the flesh that I have experienced in all the areas of my body, including my face. On several occasions the cuts were so severe that everyone who saw me following the injury insisted that I go to the emergency room for treatment and stitches. I preferred to treat myself with stevia concentrate. I simply put a few drops of stevia into the cut, and then molded the facial flesh and skin back to their correct position. If necessary, I added more stevia and held the edges of the wound together with a Band-Aid bandage or butterfly-type bandage, which I changed daily. Every time I changed the bandage, I added more stevia concentrate. My healing was much more rapid than normal and virtually pain free. Perhaps more importantly, I never experienced an infection, nor was left with any scars. With minor nicks and cuts you may not wish to bother with a bandage. The stevia concentrate will seal the wound, although it will be washed away with water.

While there is no medical research to verify this hastened healing, it does make scientific sense. Remember, stevia concentrate kills harmful bacteria by starvation, which purifies or sterilizes wounds, thus allowing your body's own healing processes to progress more efficiently and rapidly.

Please understand that I am not suggesting that you neglect getting appropriate medical treatment. I am merely reporting my own personal experiences. If you choose to experiment with stevia concentrate in this manner, begin with small cuts. This will enable you to observe the effects without endangering yourself. If you experience positive results with small scrapes and cuts, you can move on to larger cuts and abrasions. For serious wounds, of course, see your doctor.

Energy

Many people report increased energy and heightened mental concentration after ingesting stevia concentrate. This includes weight lifters, runners, and other athletes. Although this phenomenon is not well understood in relation to the average person, it is obvious for a person whose blood sugar has dropped. If the blood glucose level falls below normal, the result is a loss of energy and difficulty concentrating. If the condition is not corrected and the blood sugar continues to drop, these conditions worsen even more. The individual becomes very tired and has difficulty staying awake. If not corrected, the condition becomes extremely dangerous and can result in damage to the brain.

Wisdom suggests that people with either low or high blood sugar levels keep a bottle of stevia concentrate available at all times.

For athletes, the number of drops required to increase the energy level does not increase the body weight, as do various beverages, and therefore would not inhibit performance. Many informed weight lifters and runners, therefore, supplement with stevia concentrate.

Hair Care

One day in 1988, I received a phone call from Colonel Luís Ramirez, my Paraguayan director of operations. He had just been advised of a study conducted in Paraguay in which the subjects began to grow new hair on bald spots. The participants had shampooed their hair vigorously with a blend of a Paraguayan herbal soap containing cream of coco and stevia concentrate. According to the report, many of them grew new hair. Since I had a large bald spot on the back of my head, I anxiously tried the experiment.

Not having the combined product that was used in the study, I devised my own method. First, shampoo vigorously with a bar of Paraguayan cream of coco soap (one brand is Wisdom of the Ancients), rinsing well to eliminate any dirt, hair creme, grease, and so on. Then shampoo again, this time adding about thirty-five to forty drops of stevia concentrate to the lather. Massage your hair and scalp thoroughly and allow the lather to sit for a few minutes. After rinsing, your hair should be squeaky clean. Following a few treatments, you may find, as did I, that your hair is getting darker.

Now this was fascinating to me because my hair had been turning prematurely gray for some time. After following the procedure for a few weeks, I had a friend come up behind me and say, "Jim, what's happening to you? You've got peach fuzz on your bald spot." Of course, he had to playfully rub the spot, so that everyone around us would notice. But sure enough, it was there. I had peach fuzz. A few friends wanted to try the experiment. For some it worked extremely well. For some it was mildly successful, and others saw no change in their condition.

One of the participants had a frontal hairline that was receding significantly, which embarrassed him. Unlike the rest of us, he was *really* committed, shampooing nearly every day and leaving the combined products on his hair for a much longer period of time. He showed me his hair on a week-to-week basis because he, too, began to grow new hair. For him the growth continued until he once again had a full head of hair. He was so proud of his new hair that he had to display it to nearly everyone he met. He was actually obnoxious about it.

For me, the benefit lasted for a few years. Then my hair began to turn gray once again and to thin in the same spot. It was disappointing but I suppose that once into my sixties I should have expected it. Because I like the squeaky clean, healthy appearance of my hair, I continue to shampoo with the combination of the Paraguayan herbal soap and stevia concentrate.

Note: For men and women who use hairspray: Paraguayan herbal soap will actually break up old spray that has not been removed by other shampoos. You must shampoo and rinse several times in succession to remove this old hairspray. You will be able to feel when it is gone because your hair will no longer be sticky. Once your hair is squeaky clean, use the stevia concentrate in the final shampoo. When dry, your hair will be full bodied and beautiful. There is no end to the miracles of stevia concentrate, even if it does need a helping hand from one of its native South American sidekicks every now and then.

Mouth and Lip Sores

Numerous delighted stevia advocates have reported significant benefits regarding cracked lips, cold sores, herpes outbreaks, and mouth ulcers. Here again you may have to experience it to believe it. The concentrate seems to accelerate the healing process. As soon as you notice a lip sore or herpes outbreak, apply the concentrate, totally covering the spot on the lip. Don't wait until the next day or even a few hours. Apply the concentrate immediately. You will just naturally absorb some and lick some off, so reapply it as often as necessary. Most people say that the stevia stops the progression of the herpes dead. The soft tissue of the lip will rapidly absorb the glycoside-carrying liquid from the stevia concentrate. Perhaps, like harmful bacteria, the herpes-causing virus quickly dies of starvation, thus allowing the healing process to commence almost instantly. Those who have experienced this process say that healing is usually complete in about half the time normally expected.

Skin Care

Place a few drops of stevia concentrate on your fingertips and smooth it over your entire face. Allow it to dry and remain on your face for at least fifteen minutes. Many people leave it on for thirty to sixty minutes. Some people prefer to leave it on all night. As the liquid stevia dries, you will experience a tightening of the skin. Even after the first application, your skin will be softer to the touch and you will observe a smoothing out of the wrinkles. After several applications, you may also experience a diminishing or even a complete disappearance of various facial blemishes.

Teenagers and older people find that stevia concentrate is very helpful in controlling acne outbreaks. When you notice a pimple or other blemish, simply apply a drop of concentrate to the spot before going to bed and allow it to remain overnight. In most instances, the blemish will disappear more rapidly. Both men and women have called to say that several applications on brown age spots and warts were effective at diminishing and sometimes even eliminating them. (Note that any stains the stevia concentrate may leave on your bedlinen will come out in the wash.)

A few years ago my son Michael and I went fishing in the White Mountains of Arizona. Michael woke up one morning with an outbreak of pimples on the back of his neck. In his mid-twenties at the time, he was somewhat embarrassed. I suggested that he coat each pimple with stevia concentrate, which he did. I never take a trip, especially a camping trip, without my stevia concentrate. Its uses are just too numerous to ever be without this natural miracle.

As we were fishing, moving upstream, Michael discovered a bend in the stream where the water was deeper and moving more slowly. Just above this "hole" the land surface dropped a few feet, creating rapids and swift-moving water. This pool, at the base of the rapids, with its colder water was a natural resting and feeding area for fish. Like a restaurant in the stream, it was teaming with hungry trout. I was just a few yards downstream. When a not-so-fortunate fisherman, about seventy-five yards distant and working his way downstream, observed Michael catch two trout, he rushed to the scene. He arrived just as Michael was landing the third trout. As he threw his baited hook into the water with eager anticipation, he didn't ask, but stated, "You don't mind if I fish here with you, do you."

Perturbed at this rudeness and lack of stream etiquette, Michael turned his back slightly toward the man, bending his head downward as he gingerly removed the hook from his catch. The intruder saw the black splotches on the back of Michael's neck. His eyes got big as he stared at the unknown substance. Fear crept across his face. His thoughts were obvious: "What kind of disease is that? What if it's contagious?" He quickly pulled in his line, saying, "Uh, I think I'll try somewhere else," and departed. We enjoyed a hearty laugh, and racked up another miracle for stevia concentrate. We decided that a bottle in the pocket, for rapid application to face, neck, nose, or ears while trout fishing, might preserve productive fishing holes. Don't ever leave home without it!

Oh, yes. The pimples quickly dried up and disappeared.

Now for the big one that didn't get away—or maybe it did! I hesitate even relating these next experiences. You will understand why as you read. If you choose not to believe, your reaction will be understandable.

A friend who designs and manufactures cosmetics called to pass along her father's story, which at the time was unique. He was diagnosed with skin cancer on his head. Because both my friend and her father had experience with stevia concentrate used for other sores and blemishes, he decided to try it before submitting to surgery. He applied the concentrate daily and generously, completely covering the sore. After several days he began to notice a change in the sore's appearance. He continued the procedure. According to my friend, the sore disappeared within three to four weeks. A few years later, my friend's father and I happened to attend the same meeting. When he saw me, he came over to express his appreciation for the stevia concentrate and then stood up and related the account to all of the people at the large gathering. He said his cancer had never returned.

The owner of a health food store in California telephoned because one of his customers wanted to talk with me. The man just wanted to say thank you. He told me of the cancer that had appeared on his head. He, too, tried the concentrate before submitting to surgery. He said that within a few weeks the sore had disappeared.

A highly respected attorney, now retired, called me to request that I develop a special cream to treat skin cancer. He had been the patent attorney for a number of pharmaceutical companies and possessed significant scientific knowledge of, and experience with, the wonderful healing benefits of lapacho (pau d'arco). He had also studied several research documents concerning stevia and had reasoned that the two herbs, along with a few others he had in mind, would, in his words, "cure" the skin cancer that had appeared on his head. In fact, he sent me some scientific research documents on both stevia and lapacho that I had not previously read.

While I agreed with his theory, I explained that I could not make and market a product to treat cancer. Even if it worked 100 percent of the time, it would lead to my arrest, and possibly even incarceration, which he knew. I guess desperate people are willing to take desperate measures, however, especially with someone else's freedom. Regardless of how effective a product (and in this case, a specially designed medicine) might be, it must first be approved by the FDA before it can be sold to consumers (now called patients), and prescribed by medical doctors. That, according to the most recent estimates by the pharmaceutical industry, costs $500 million to $700 million and takes five to ten years of research and trials. These figures may have been exaggerated by the pharmaceutical firms for political purposes and pricing justification but they enable us to understand the extraordinarily high cost of bringing a new drug to market. This is why the pharmaceutical industry is reserved for multibillion-dollar companies.

The attorney then requested that I make the cream just for him. My response, of course, was that I could not sustain the expense of creating a product for only one person, especially if it took just one or two units of the product to effect a cure. However, I told him that I would speak with my skincare product designer and see if she would make the product for him. (This was not the same lady I referred to in the previous account.) I told him that he would have to bear the entire expense but that I would provide the raw materials at no cost. Luckily, my skincare product designer agreed to the endeavor. I called the attorney back and told him, adding that he would need to pay the product designer in advance, to which he readily agreed. The attorney then said, "Jim, I don't understand why you're not willing to make this product. I know it'll be effective. You don't have to sell it as a cancer cure. I'll tell people that I know who have skin cancer and the word will spread like wildfire."

My response was straightforward: "I don't doubt its potential effectiveness. Your idea is excellent. It's just not necessary."

His query was rapid fire: "What do you mean 'not necessary'?"

My answer was simple: "Because I think that stevia concentrate would be every bit as effective at a fraction of the cost. You already have some. Why don't you try it before going to all this trouble and expense?"

A few weeks later I began to wonder if the attorney had followed through with the arrangement. I called my skincare product designer and asked if she had completed the project. She said that he had never called. My next phone call was to the attorney. "Jim," he said, "I decided to try your suggestion first. You were right. It worked. There was no need to make another product."

Now, as exciting as these stories are, no scientific documentation exists to back them up. I cannot prove that they were true experiences, nor would I ever attempt to do so. They are, as medical professionals say, "only anecdotal." Which apparently means that despite the effectiveness of a product on humans, if it was not discovered and tested by the scientific community, and "proven" in scientific studies, it does not qualify as an acceptable product. However, I spent most of my youth in the blazing sun of the Arizona summers, shirtless and hatless. Even now, my wife is always after me because I do my yard work in the summer sun, usually without a hat. My fair skin always burns easily and severely. I suspect that I have had thousands of sunburns on my forehead and, when I was young, on my back. When the sores appear, I have found that applying stevia concentrate for two to three weeks totally eliminates them, leaving only fresh new skin.

Please be aware that I am not recommending that anyone with skin cancer try this. Cancer is dangerous, and its consequences can be fatal. I am simply relating experiences of my own or reported to me by others. If you choose to try stevia concentrate in this manner, you do so at your own risk. If some improvement is not evident within two or three weeks, you should immediately return to your physician for treatment. In addition, you should openly discuss any experiments with your physician, who could then monitor the results. You, as the consumer/patient, would have to take all the responsibility and agree to hold the doctor harmless regardless of the outcome.

Sore Throat

If you have a sore throat, place two or more dropperfuls (with about thirty-five to forty drops per dropper) of stevia concentrate in the back of your mouth. Tilt your head so that when you swallow the liquid, it will pass over and coat the area of your throat that is sore. Within thirty to sixty seconds you should experience a significant reduction in the soreness. This process may completely eliminate the pain for several hours. When you first feel the irritation begin to return, repeat the process. You can repeat this procedure as often as needed, but in most instances, the pain will not return after only two or three applications. Stevia concentrate is exceptionally effective at reducing pain. Perhaps, it also reduces the viral count due to its natural zinc content. It may also be that viruses, like bacteria and humans, cannot digest the sweet glycosides. No conclusive scientific research has been done on this phenomenon but one positive experience is more impressive than a thousand written words either in favor of or against the procedure.

Recently, a large Arizona chain of health food stores opened a new store in Mesa. To attract customers, it held a product exhibit under a large, open-sided tent in the parking lot of the shopping mall. My company was asked to participate. This chain did not carry all of our products, including our dark stevia concentrate. We hoped for an opportunity to visit with a corporate executive during the exhibit. As fortune would dictate, the corporate vice president of purchasing, with whom we had not been able to obtain an appointment, came to us. He said, "One of my managers has a terrible sore throat. Do you have anything that would give her a little relief?"

"Yes, we do," I responded. "Bring her over and I'll show her how to use it."

Within a few moments the vice president returned with the young lady. I handed her the bottle of stevia concentrate and told her what to do. "Your sore throat will be gone in thirty seconds," I said, suggesting to the vice president that he time her. They looked at each other like I was totally out of my mind, but she swallowed two dropperfuls of stevia concentrate and he timed out thirty seconds. Astounded, the young lady exclaimed, "My sore throat is gone!" I gave her the bottle of stevia, and he gave my vice president of marketing an appointment.

I have used stevia concentrate in this manner for several years. It is always fun to suggest the procedure to someone suffering with a sore throat. People have become so brainwashed by the pharmaceutical and medical industries that we doubt that any natural, multiuse substance can cause such rapid healing—and at such a small cost. Wait until you see the faces of these doubting Thomases and Janes as the soreness disappears within seconds. It makes you feel like politely doffing your white hat, mounting your trusty steed, shouting "Hi Ho Silver!," and riding away into the sunset. Another suffering soul rescued—without having to fire a silver bullet. On second thought, maybe that was a "silver bullet," and the triumphant shout should be "Hi Ho Stevia!"

Water Retention

Along with all of the benefits discussed above, stevia also acts as a natural but gentle diuretic. An overabundance of liquid in the body increases weight, physical fatigue, and blood pressure, while decreasing mental ability and efficient digestion. Stevia assists the body in eliminating excess body fluids.

In these last two chapters, we have discussed the forms of stevia that are as natural as fruits and vegetables. As man has found many ways of preparing produce, so have we found various ways of offering stevia: fresh and dried leaves, ground dried leaves, leaves cooked into a sauce, and the sauce then dried again and pressed into tablets. In the next chapter, we will discuss stevioside and the various forms in which it is sold to the consumer. All of these forms of stevia are high in nutritional value and perform vital functions both within and upon the human body.

5

A Superior, High-Intensity Sweetener: Stevioside

"A Turkish study has revealed that as we get older, sugar doesn't taste as sweet—and 45% of women report that they start eating sweeter foods as a result. Switching to sugar substitutes can help; they're up to 600 times sweeter than sugar, with fewer calories."

—From *Woman's World*, July 29, 2003

Since the discovery of stevioside, food scientists in several countries have been laboring to prove its safety for humans and to develop uses for stevia's incredible sweetening power. Stevioside is the form of stevia that is 250 to 300 times sweeter than sugar and has been used in foods in Japan since the early 1970s. Today China, followed by Korea, probably produces the greatest amount of stevioside. The sugar industry and especially the artificial sweetener industry have done everything in their power to keep this form of stevia out of the United States.

We will thoroughly analyze several scientific studies in upcoming chapters that will help you draw your own conclusions about the safety of stevia as compared to aspartame. You can then make your own comparison to the natural and artificial sweeteners currently in our food supply. For now, simply accept the fact that in all of these years, and after consuming the hundreds of tons of stevioside used to sweeten foods, there has never been a reported or documented incident of harm to man or beast caused by the normal ingestion of stevia or stevioside.

PURE STEVIOSIDE PRODUCTS

We live in a world of processed foods that are filled with sweeteners carrying various names. Without these high-calorie and high-glycemic-index sweeteners, the food products would not sell because they would taste bad. The result is that we ingest more high-calorie foods and sweeteners that are rapidly converted into glucose than our bodies can utilize. Because we eat too many of these foods plus don't move our bodies enough, we store fat. Scientists and consumers who have studied and used stevioside believe that it is the most logical and safest answer to this troubling dilemma.

Stevia Extract Powder

Most of the manufacturers currently marketing stevioside to the public call it stevia extract powder. Stevia extract powder is intensely sweet because it consists of the various sweet glycosides extracted from stevia leaves by patented processes. Its color is semiwhite to white. It contains no calories and no carbohydrates. The intensity of its sweetness and its aftertaste depend upon the ratio of the various glycosides to one another and the product's purity. In most instances, the greater the content of rebaudioside A, the less noticeable the aftertaste and the more intense the sweetness. However, this is not a hard-and-fast rule and may not always hold true owing to the various techniques used for extraction and processing. As with the old cliché about pudding, the proof of the stevia (whether whole-leaf or extract powder) is in the tasting.

Stevia leaves normally have a very low content of rebaudioside A, which is 400 times sweeter than sugar. However in recent years, botanists have developed plants with a significantly increased amount of both steviosides and rebaudioside A. They have accomplished this with cross-pollination, using honeybees. Also, food scientists have discovered that when certain enzymes are added, stevioside can be converted into rebaudioside A, thus increasing the sweet taste while diminishing the aftertaste. Whether or not this enzyme action affects the safety of the product is unknown, but unlikely.

Stevia extract powder is available primarily in health food stores under several different brand names. However, many of the regional and national supermarket and drug store chains now also offer products. The quality, the content of rebaudioside A, and thus the final taste will vary in the different brands. Look for brands that are standardized to 90 percent or higher in steviosides. What this means is that the product is 90 percent steviosides and rebaudiosides and 10 percent other constituents of the stevia leaf. A product that is 80 percent stevioside is generally regarded as food grade and 90 percent or better as pharmaceutical grade. The quality and the sweet taste of a product standardized to a minimum of 90 percent steviosides are significantly better than those of a product that is less than this. Also, the higher the content of rebaudioside A, the sweeter the product, and the better the taste. When the label indicates that the product is standardized to a minimum of 90 percent steviosides and 40 percent rebaudioside A, it means that of the 90 percent steviosides, 40 percent is rebaudioside A.

The cost of producing a product that is standardized to 90 percent steviosides, of which 40 percent is rebaudioside A, is greater than that for a product with a lesser content. Rebaudioside A of 60 percent to 80 percent can be achieved but the cost to the manufacturer and thus the resulting sales price to the consumer will be significantly higher. The increased sweetness may not be worth the increased cost. It is important to read the labels of the various brands. If you compare only the prices, you may be disappointed in the quality of the product you choose and thus its ability to sweeten foods and beverages. This can be critical when baking or cooking. A higher priced product may be far less expensive in the long run. Stevia extract powders that have a rebaudioside A content of 60 percent to 80 percent are primarily for food and beverage manufacturers.

Uses

Stevia extract powder is excellent for both cooking and baking. (Aspartame cannot be used for cooking, since it breaks down when exposed to heat.) Usually about one-fourth to one-third of a teaspoon will replace a full cup of sugar. (For a stevia conversion chart, see Appendix A.) This will vary depending on what you are sweetening, and the brand you are using, so you will need to experiment. Different brands are anywhere from 200 to 300 times sweeter than sugar. Remember when substituting that you will need to replace the bulk lost when the sugar or other alternative sweetener is removed with another ingredient. In addition, one form of the stevia may be more desirable than another form in a specific recipe. There are several fine stevia cookbooks available to assist beginners. (For a list of cookbooks, see Appendix B.)

Which form of stevia you decide upon and how you use it will be determined by your own personal objective. If you are diabetic or hypoglycemic, you may wish to use stevia extract powder, clear liquid, or stevia concentrate. Baked goods made with stevia extract powder will not have exactly the same sweet taste as pastries made with sugar or honey. This is because of the basic difference between stevia and sugar and also because the sugar bulk must be replaced by an increased amount of flour, applesauce, or another filler. However, the taste is quite acceptable, and most diabetics and nutritionists agree that it is better than that of the other alternative sweeteners available.

If your goal is simply to reduce the number of calories or amount of conventional sweeteners in your diet but maintain a specific sweet taste, you may prefer to blend stevia extract powder with another natural sweetener such as sugar, honey, or fructose. A small amount of stevia combined with these sweeteners will maintain the taste you are used to while significantly reducing the calories. For instructions on blending stevia with other sweeteners, see any of the cookbooks listed in Appendix B.

It is this pure white powder form of stevia that many manufacturers of toothpastes and mouthwashes would like to add to their products. Unlike stevia concentrate, this extract will not discolor the product. The bacteria that cause the various gum diseases and tooth decay ingest the stevioside but are unable to digest it, so many die, thus reducing the size of their colonies. The result is improved oral hygiene, including fewer cavities and less plaque. Unfortunately, the FDA has banned the use of stevia, in any of its forms in toothpaste and has issued orders in the form of import alerts for any toothpaste containing it imported into the United States to be confiscated and destroyed. Fortunately, the FDA has not yet invaded the bathrooms of Americans to see if we add stevia ourselves to our toothpaste or mouthwash.

Stevia extract powder is also the form of stevia used in Asia and South America in numerous commercial soft drinks, candies, chewing gums, soy sauce, ice creams and sherbets, frozen foods, fruit and citrus juices, and low-calorie foods—as well as toothpaste. This is because, as determined by all research, stevia contains no calories and has a glycemic index of zero. This means that stevia is not converted to glucose in the human body and does not contribute to fat creation or storage. Imagine for a moment the improvement that will result in the weight and overall health and well-being of Americans when the FDA finally permits stevia to be used in candies, ice cream, pastries, soft drinks, juices, and other beverages. Your favorite sweet desserts and beverages can have 75 to 80 percent fewer calories, plus will improve your oral hygiene while you eat or drink them.

This begs the question: Is it the FDA that is ultimately responsible for the fact that more than 60 percent of Americans are overweight? Why are certain FDA executives so adamant about preventing the unrestricted use of stevia by Americans? Is it simply because stevia was introduced into this country by small herbal companies and not the pharmaceutical giants? The huge drug companies seem to have no problems getting their *artificial* sweeteners approved—even when the bulk of the scientific research has proven the sweeteners to be harmful to humans and, in the case of a few, to actually cause weight gain. (See Chapters 6 and 9.)

Stevia extract powder is not recommended for sweetening beverages by the glass or cup because it is difficult to measure an amount small enough. Also, it is a very light powder, making it difficult to dissolve, especially in a cold drink. You would need to wet a toothpick, touch the stevia extract, and then stir the powder sticking to the toothpick into your drink. For this reason clear liquid stevia extract and stevia tablets have been developed.

Clear Liquid Stevia Extract

Clear liquid stevia extract is made by blending stevioside (stevia extract powder) with pure water. A preservative, such as grapefruit seed extract, must be added to prevent spoiling. If the product comes with a dropper, care should be taken not to touch the tip to other foods or items, including your fingers. This would contaminate the dropper tip, resulting in the introduction of germs into the solution when the dropper is replaced. This form of stevia does not have the same bacteria-inhibiting power as dark stevia concentrate. The stevioside will sometimes separate from the water and appear as white flakes floating in the solution. If the flakes disappear with vigorous shaking, the product is all right. If the flakes remain, the product may be too old and should be discarded.

Some manufacturers use alcohol instead of water to make clear liquid stevia extract. While alcohol acts as an effective preservative, it alters the taste of the product. In addition, an alcohol-based product is not as sweet as a water-based product, and also not as healthy.

Clear liquid stevia extract made with water should always be refrigerated after opening.

Uses

Like all the other forms of stevia, clear liquid stevia extract is safe for both diabetics and hypoglycemics. It is a preferable sweetener for people trying to lose fat or maintain a desired weight. Because it is mixed with water, it is not as intensely sweet as stevia extract powder.

Clear liquid stevia extract is a remarkable sweetener for lemonade and other citrus drinks. It is an excellent sweetener for any beverage that needs the sweet taste of health. Try it on cereal (added to the milk) and in hot and cold chocolate milk, fruit juices, soft drinks, soups, pasta sauces, and any liquid foods. A few drops added to the water used to cook vegetables will give the veggies a sweeter flavor. Because you can make the vegetables as sweet as desired, without adding calories, children may eat them without complaint.

There are numerous health beverages being sold today that may be good for the body but taste awful. Adding several drops of clear liquid stevia extract will make them much more palatable, even if the drink is an aloe vera beverage. Add a few drops to toothpaste to improve oral hygiene. Clear liquid stevia extract is convenient and does not alter the color of foods or drinks. Simply start with a few drops, taste, and add more until you achieve your preferred taste profile.

Stevia Tablets

Stevia tablets consist of stevia extract powder pressed into tiny white tablets bound together with fillers such as cornstarch, lactose, and modified cellulose gum. Each tablet has the sweetening equivalent of one teaspoon of sugar. The tablets dissolve quickly in both hot and cold beverages, although they do take a few seconds longer to do so in cold beverages.

Uses

Stevia tablets are designed specifically for sweetening beverages. They are convenient for travel and for carrying in the pocket or purse to restaurants, coffee shops, and the homes of friends. The measurement is precise—one tiny tablet replaces a teaspoon of sugar.

BLENDED STEVIOSIDE PRODUCTS

When Congress enacted the Dietary Supplement Health and Education Act of 1994 (signed by President Clinton on October 25, 1994), no one knew if the FDA would permit stevia to be included under the Act. Even if it was allowed, there was little good-quality stevia or stevioside available to be imported into and sold in the United States. We were well into 1995 when the FDA decided that it would not prevent stevia and stevioside products from being sold as dietary or nutritional supplements, or used as an ingredients in such products. It was adamant, however, that no form of stevia should be used as a sweetening ingredient in another product or sold to the consuming public as a sweetener. Had the FDA really had evidence that stevia was or could be harmful, it could have prevented its use as a nutritional supplement. As of this writing, stevia has again been in use in the United States for nine years without, to my knowledge, a single report of harm or any adverse effect upon anyone.

Following stevia's approval as a dietary or nutritional supplement, friendly competitors called me to discuss how to resolve the supply problem. What little stevioside was available would have to be blended with a carrier in order to function as a product for consumers. Also, we felt it was a good idea to create a consumer-friendly product that could be compared to and replace sugar in a measurable manner. We discussed various potential carriers available at the time, including maltodextrin, maltodextrose, fructose, and lactose.

Stevia products that include these carriers may be used to sweeten or improve the flavor of nearly any food or drink. Use the stevia product just as you use sugar or any artificial sweetener. While stevia is calorie-free and has a glycemic index of zero, *these carriers do have calories and a low-to-high glycemic index.* When making a choice, remember that the higher the glycemic index, the faster the body converts the substance into glucose, so it is important to read the label and take note of all the ingredients before making a selection. Also, each of these carriers will result in a different flavor profile. If you find the taste of one formulation objectionable, or if for some reason you can't use one, try another.

Stevioside and Maltodextrin

For much of the population, maltodextrin is an acceptable choice as a carrier in stevia products because it has been affirmed by the FDA that it is GRAS as a direct human food ingredient. It is used as a bulking agent in numerous processed foods because it dissolves easily and is relatively nonhygroscopic (does not absorb moisture out of the air). It is an easy product to manufacture and is inexpensive. However, it is made from cornstarch and is a complex carbohydrate containing dextrose, maltose, maltotriose, and higher saccharides. It is a mild, bland-flavored sugar. Maltodextrins are used in a wide variety of reduced- and full-calorie foods, and are often used as a means of carbohydrate loading in specialized food applications. This is the bulking agent often used in non-nutritive artificial sweeteners such as Equal and NutraSweet. Obviously, this is not the best bulking agent for products designed for people who have a blood sugar problem or who want to lose weight or maintain a specific weight. This blend, sometimes modified with other ingredients, is now available under several brand names, including NOW Foods, Stevita, and Kal. Actual product names, however, differ.

Uses

Stevioside and maltodextrin blends may be used the same way any sugar or artificial sweetener is with foods and beverages. Unlike chemical sweeteners, this blend can be used in cooking and baking. The taste profiles of the different products vary but all are generally acceptable. If one brand does not meet your taste preference, try another.

Stevioside and Inulin

In 1994 there were only about three suppliers of stevia to the United States market. The others decided to use one or more of the stevioside and maltodextrin blends as their carrier of choice with a small amount of stevioside. They packaged and sold their new products in either small bottles or single-serving paper packets. Thus, they created products similar to those then being marketed to consumers in Asia and South America. The problem was that the carriers used were all sweeteners and not completely safe for diabetics—and the early combinations did not taste very good. However, healthwise, the products were superior to the artificial sweeteners that were then available in stores. Even so, I was concerned that the FDA, in what I believe were its attempts to protect the territory of aspartame, NutraSweet, and Equal, would declare that these new products were sweeteners and not nutritional supplements and then remove them from the market. We chose to market only whole-leaf stevia products and pure stevia extract powder, all of which were clearly acceptable under the regulations.

Since all products utilizing stevioside as an ingredient were to be labeled and sold only as nutritional supplements, we wanted to comply strictly with the regulation and have an absolutely truthful label. I called my son Steve (the one people continue to believe stevia is named after), who had just completed his active duty in the Army, into my office, discussed the problem, and gave him the assignment to find "the perfect carrier" for stevioside. The requirements we decided upon were:

- It had to be white and mildly sweet.

- It had to be good for the human body.

- It had to be officially classified as a dietary or nutritional supplement.

- It had to blend well with stevioside—and it had to taste good!

- The end product had to be a true nutritional supplement that tasted like a sweetener.

- It had to dissolve quickly and be easy to use.

- It had to be completely safe for diabetics and hypoglycemics.

- It had to have a zero to very low glycemic index.

- It had to contain zero to very few calories.

The task was not easy. It took a full year and we lost a year of market penetration. Everyone thought that I was foolish to wait, but integrity and honor are determined neither by profits won nor lost.

At the end of a year of diligent searching, Steve came into my office and excitedly exclaimed, "Dad, I've found it!" He handed me the research and use data on fructooligosaccharides (FOS), a form of inulin that was being introduced as a functional food. Perhaps you will remember that stevia leaves contain two compounds of inulin. FOS was the perfect product to blend with stevioside. It is a product of nature, existing in thousands of plants, including fruits and vegetables. It is white, mildly sweet, dissolves readily, and is officially classified as a nutritional supplement. Like stevia, it is stable in both heat and a low pH. Also, it is a prebiotic, meaning that its primary function within the human body is to feed (nourish and strengthen) the friendly flora in the small intestine and colon. These are the bacteria that must flourish in your gut if you are to be healthy. Inulin is their preferred food supply. Inulin is also a soluble fiber. (For more on the benefits of inulin, see below and page 103.)

This was Steve's project and he carried it to a very successful completion. However, the precise blend was not easy to achieve. It took another year of research, of trial and error, before we learned how to blend the two different-sized particles together to form a superior product. We were then two years behind our competitors. But the wait was worth it. Many dieticians and nutritionists agree that Steve's SteviaPlus Fiber is one of the most incredible stevia products available today and recommend it in their articles and books. This new creation of a sweet prebiotic nutritional supplement was rapidly accepted by consumers and is currently the most widely accepted stevia product in America. Hospital dieticians, not affiliated with the FDA or AMA, are counseling diabetic and overweight patients to use this stevia-inulin sweetener instead of sugar and artificial sweeteners. Hospitals are even considering offering it on food service trays, replacing artificial sweeteners.

❧ The Benefits of Inulin

Inulin is a naturally occurring constituent in more than 36,000 plants worldwide. Many of these plants are fruits and vegetables, including bananas, tomatoes, onions, asparagus, Jerusalem artichoke, garlic, leeks, and chicory, which are a part of the traditional human diet. Inulin, containing natural fructooligosaccharides (FOS), is the energy reserve in these plants.

Inulin is a prebiotic—that is, it nourishes the good bacteria in the intestinal tract. While inulin is a carbohydrate, it is not digestible by the human body. It passes essentially unaltered through the stomach and small intestines directly to the beneficial bacteria, which reside in the large intestine, or colon. In addition, inulin is 100 percent clear and soluble dietary fiber.

Soluble fiber is essential for good health. One of the major weaknesses of many of the currently popular diets is a lack of natural fiber. Anyone on a reduced-carbohydrate diet such as Dr. Atkins', Protein Power, or The Zone should take supplemental inulin daily.

What are other benefits of ingesting inulin? After inulin reaches the colon, it is fermented by microflora that produce various metabolic end products of nutritional significance. By feeding these beneficial microflora, it also helps them to multiply, reducing the space available for detrimental microflora. In a nutshell and in common everyday terms, studies have shown that as these beneficial bacteria increase in the colon, they provide the body with the following benefits:

- They cleanse the colon and improve regularity.
- They produce vitamins that are essential for health and well-being.
- They strengthen the immune system.
- They support the health of the liver, and thus its ability to function.
- They prevent the overgrowth of Candida, a yeast, and a host of harmful bacteria including *E. coli* and salmonella.
- They help control the formation of free radicals.
- They do not adversely affect the blood sugar.

In order to really appreciate what inulin does for the human body, you need to understand what well-nourished, flourishing colonies of good bacteria do for the human body—for *your* body. Without them you cannot be healthy.

Uses

SteviaPlus can be used exactly like sugar and any chemical artificial sweetener, including NutraSweet, Equal, Sweet n' Low, and Splenda. It can be used in cooking and baking and in frozen foods and beverages, including coffee, teas, and juices. It is not formulated to be eaten out of the hand like sugar, but once it is put into a beverage or onto grapefruit, fruit, cereal, and other foods, it offers a deliciously sweet flavor. It is about ten times sweeter than sugar, so when cooking or baking with it, remember to begin with already developed recipes. (For a list of recommended cookbooks, see Appendix B.)

Strange New Names

The herbal and holistic industry has struggled to invent new terms to define the nutritious foods and herbs that were designed by nature (I prefer to credit God) to nourish the entire human organism. These newly coined terms had to be combinations of words not yet banned by the FDA. Thus, we see the evolution of descriptive vocabulary, with words such as phytochemicals, nutraceuticals, phytoceuticals, phytonutraceuticals, and the less technical term, functional foods.

These words are intended to help the public understand that the total constituency of naturally occurring nutrients within herbs and foods are designed not only to feed but also to stimulate health, vitality, and healing within the human body. The concept is simple: Constantly feed the body the nutrients it requires, in the form designed specifically for it, thus, allowing the body to absorb and assimilate what it needs and discard the remainder. With the needed nutrients, the body may well have the ability to heal itself—without harmful, overly powerful debilitating drugs. Within its own corporeal being, each human body possesses more intelligence concerning its own specific internal needs than do all the scientists and doctors now living combined.

As consumer demand increases for the nutritional, health, and sweetening benefits of stevia products, these products are beginning to appear in supermarket and drugstore chains. Ask for them. Search for them—but not on the sweetener shelf. The FDA will not permit them to be next to or compared with sweeteners or artificial sweeteners. Just as well. I believe those products are harmful to the human body. Stevia is not. Store managers place stevia products in various locations, so save time and ask the manager to show you where they are. When you do this, you will also let him or her know that there is a demand for stevia. The benefits you will receive from the best stevia products are well worth the search. Discovering the "right" stevia products for you or your loved one, can be to your health and well-being what discovering a diamond mine or oil well in your own back yard would be to your economic health.

Stevia has become a true blessing in the lives of millions of North Americans. But introducing stevia to the citizens of the United States has been a most difficult and dangerous endeavor. When the project was commenced in 1982, I had no concept of the dangers that lay ahead, to both my physical and financial well-being. A well-intentioned but unwise statement or a wrong decision could have put me in a filthy dungeon in Paraguay, or in a United States prison. For years I would teeter on the edge of financial ruin—all because of my belief in the wonderful healing and sweetening benefits of stevia and my determination to bring it to Americans.

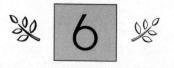

Stevia, Aspartame, and Fat Storage

"Cells get both chemical and electrical information from their surroundings . . . [and] also pass soluble chemicals back and forth from one to another through gaps or channels in their cell membranes. When those channels and their messages are blocked, embryo cells develop defects, which suggest that losing those messages lets their genetic processes get off track."

—Dean Black, Ph.D., *Health at the Crossroads*
(Tapestry Press, 1988)

When your cells are bathed in harmful chemicals and pollutants, they cannot function properly and must mutate or die. Their information and response systems are impeded, they cannot receive the nutrients they require and as a result cannot maintain their correct nutrient ratio, and they are unable to eliminate their waste products. The purity of the fluid surrounding a cell is crucial to the cell's ability to function and survive. Even further, a small loss of this fluid or change in its concentration of electrolytes can kill us. Therefore, maintaining this fluid composition, in content, balance, and context, is critical.

Stevioside extracts are totally natural, coming from plant leaves, and are not assimilated into the human body but passed unchanged through the intestines in solid fecal waste. Because steviosides do not enter our cells, they neither interrupt, alter the context of, nor impede cellular function. Apparently, they simply have no effect whatsoever upon the structure or function of our cells.

Fat storage is multifaceted and the result of numerous interruptions and chemical alterations within the cellular structure and function of the human body. Your brain is the caretaker of your whole body. It controls and maintains every process and function of it. Every gland, organ, tissue, and cell is in communication with and regulated by it. Your brain's primary function is to maintain your body in the best state of health that you will permit, based on what you allow to enter your body and mind through the various pathways. Every other function of your brain is subservient to maintaining your health, your well-being, and, most importantly, your survival.

HUNGER SATIATION AND WASTE ELIMINATION MECHANISMS

Hunger is far more complex than stomach emptiness and the associated pangs of the resultant contractions. Stomach contractions cease when glucose is injected into the bloodstream, even when the stomach is totally empty. The metabolic factors of the body relate the feeling of hunger to the maintenance of energy, which is governed by the presence of glucose, carbohydrates, and fats available for immediate burning. However, as Dr. Tobin Watkinson informed us in Chapter 4, the signal pathway between the hypothalamus and the stomach must function correctly during the process of eating in order to turn off hunger once the stomach is satiated.

Also, in our modern lifestyle we tend to eat too fast, gulping our food down so we can get to the movie or somewhere else on time. We eat while watching television and have little or no conversation, which would in itself slow down the procedure. Thus, we allow our body little time to process our food into glucose and to communicate satiation, or because our focus is on other activities, we simply do not receive the satiation transmission. Simply stated, we put too much food on our plates, we eat too fast, and we continue to gorge ourselves even after we are satiated. Then we sit, expending no energy. We don't walk to our destinations, we ride, and upon arrival, we sit. Young people rarely go outside after a meal and play physically active, energy-burning games. They sit and play computer games. Energy consumed in the form of food but unexpended either by maintaining bodily processes, burning in the muscles, or wasting by brown adipose tissue (special fat-burning cells) results in fat storage leading to obesity.

Durk Pearson and Sandy Shaw, in their book *Life Extension,* offer this counsel:

> When you eat, pay attention to your eating! You feel full and stop eating because your brain releases CCK [cholecystokinin] hormone. What you think and what you perceive controls this release, NOT the number of calories consumed. Eliminate distractions while you're eating. Turn off the TV or radio. Put down that newspaper. Pay close attention to the aroma, taste, mouth feel, and appearance of your food. It's fun! Eat slowly and deliberately. You will be amazed at how little food it takes to fill and satisfy you if you pay very close attention to your eating. If you eat slowly, you give your hypothalamus time to release CCK and make you feel full. If you wolf your food down, you will consume far more calories than are necessary for complete satiation, due to the delay for CCK release.[1]

All living organisms that take in fuel must of necessity release waste products. So it is with the human body—from each cell to the entire organism. When waste, pollutants, toxins, and pathogens cannot be eliminated from the body in a timely manner, disease and eventual death are certain. Therefore, the body has several pathways of elimination, all controlled by the brain. Bodily waste, toxic materials, bacteria, and viruses are expelled via the colon and urinary tract. We eliminate toxins, pollutants, and pathogens through our sweat glands (especially under the arms) and tear ducts, and by sneezing and coughing. When necessary, our brain kills viruses and bacteria by increasing our body temperature through fever and also directs the colon to expel harmful materials and organisms through diarrhea. To obstruct or prevent any of these natural processes of elimination from occurring is foolish and will, in time, result in serious consequences in the ability of our body to function properly.

THERMOGENESIS AND OUR SET POINT FOR BODY FAT

The brain maintains body temperature by a system of thermometer neurons located in the hypothalamus, which monitor blood temperature. If there is a variance of about 1°C (1.8°F) from the correct set point of 37°C (98.6°F), the neurons alter the rate of firing, which triggers actions within the body designed either to cool or warm the blood. Cooling is achieved by releasing fluid through sweating and vasodilation (widening of the diameter of the blood vessels) in the arms, legs, and head, thus increasing heat loss. Warming is accomplished by increasing muscle tone and by shivering, and also by curling up the body, thus constricting blood vessels in the skin, which reduces heat loss.[2] Heat is also produced in the body as energy and is expended through the process of thermogenesis. The word *thermogenesis* means "heat creation." *Thermo* means "heat," and *genesis* means "creation."

Because the combination of overeating and underexercising is the bane of our times, we need to understand the hunger mechanism, caloric utilization, and waste elimination processes better. We will then also better comprehend why the processes (seemingly miracles) that we have discussed in this book so far occurred after adding various forms of stevia to the diet. While it is important to govern our calorie consumption, we now understand that gaining and losing fat is not simply a process of caloric intake versus output, or "energy in, energy out." A calorie is a unit of heat, which is also energy. One calorie is the amount of heat energy required to raise the temperature of 1 gram of water by 1°C. It takes a brisk thirty-minute walk to burn off 300 calories, and it takes 365 days of brisk walking to burn off thirty-five pounds of fat.

The accumulation of white fat is the body's method of storing energy (during times of perceived plenty) for future use. When the brain perceives that a time of food shortage or famine is coming, it alerts the body to begin filling up its storage units with fat, and to manufacture and fill up new fat cells, to provide energy during those future days of deprivation.

A fascinating corollary to this is the Old Testament story of Joseph, son of the Prophet Jacob, who was sold by his brothers into slavery in Egypt. As a result of his good works, wisdom, and guidance by God, he rose to be second in authority to Pharaoh by correctly interpreting dreams given to Pharaoh by God. Pharaoh had dreamed that seven very fat but well-developed and muscular kine (cattle) came up out of the Nile River (water) and fed themselves in the meadows (or marshland) near the river. They were followed by seven more kine coming up out of the river, but these latter kine were very "ill favored and leanfleshed" such as had never been seen in Egypt. The seven lean kine ate the seven fat kine but put on no weight by eating them. The Pharaoh also dreamed of seven ears of grain being produced on one stock. This is unusual because all the grains except corn produce only one ear per stock. While corn produces two ears, it did not grow in Egypt. Then, apparently upon the same stock, grew seven ears of grain that were "withered, thin, and blasted by the east wind," which was a very hot, dry, and destructive wind. The seven withered ears of grain devoured the seven well-formed ears.

Joseph understood that the seven fat kine and the seven normal ears of grain represented seven years of plenty that would be followed by seven years of severe famine, represented by the lean kine and withered ears of grain. During the years of famine, little grain or grass would be available for man or beast. There would be seven years of abundant rainfall at the upper waters of the Nile River, resulting in the annual flooding of the Nile, which would deposit its mineral-rich soils upon the farmland that bordered the river, helping to produce excellent, abundant, and highly nutritious crops. However, this would be followed by seven years of drought during which the waters of the Nile not only would not flood, but would also severely recede. Thus, the drought condition would provide increasingly less water for irrigation and production of the mineral-rich soil for plant growth and development, resulting in each harvest being poorer than the previous one. The correlation between the dream messages and our own bodily function is that in preparation for a coming period of famine the bodies of animals store extra amounts of fat. Even though the hungry and lean kine and the withered and thin ears of grain devoured their more abundant counterparts to store energy in preparation for the lean years, they stored no fat but expended it all in survival.

In the Biblical story, Joseph, being inspired by God, understood that the way to survive the drought-caused famine was to store grain for the future energy needs and survival of both man and beast. So Pharaoh put Joseph in charge of all Egypt and he ordered the construction of storehouses in which vast quantities of grain (stored energy) could be housed. This permitted the people to continue to purchase and eat grain in relatively normal amounts. Thus, in the time of famine the people drew energy from the fat cells (storehouses) accumulated in times of plenty, but did not add to the fat stores in their bodies.[3]

THE BRAIN AND LIVER: A DYNAMIC DUO

The currently prevailing concept of caloric storage is that the brain, when functioning correctly, regulates body fat gain and loss around a set point, and utilizes various means to maintain it. When functioning properly, the hypothalamus controls appetite and the absorption of nutrients into the body. It also regulates metabolism and, thus, caloric expenditure. Because the most fundamental function of the brain is to ensure survival, it is programmed to hold energy in reserve. When we are young, we are physically active, constantly taxing the energy reserves of our body. The more active we are in demanding energy from our body, the harder our brain works to provide that energy. The brain understands the life equation that constant energy demand with unequaled energy input results in the depletion of energy reserves through the burning of stored fat, and then muscle tissue, resulting in the wasting and eventual death of the body. Thus, even when we reduce our energy output, our brain, having been programmed by our prior demand, continues to store energy in the form of fat. We exacerbate the situation when we continue to eat the same amount of food (calories) required for our former energy output.

Fat deposits are created when many single units of fatty acids are linked together. When we need to draw on these stored fatty acids for energy, they are broken down. Each gram of fat provides nine calories of energy, while each gram of protein or glucose provides only four calories of energy. Some researchers suggest that this is the reason we are less hungry when we burn our fat stores for energy.

The liver is the organ responsible for the cleansing and detoxification of the body. It does this by filtering the blood supply and eliminating waste through the colon and kidneys. When the liver becomes congested or overloaded with toxic material, the entire system becomes susceptible to toxin infiltration, with disease or diseaselike systems resulting. Some toxins are normally generated by the metabolic processes of cellular elimination and are generally excreted without problems. However, the toxins that result when we eat, drink, or breathe non-natural substances can upset the functions of the brain and the preset processes and responses of the glands and organs of the body and may not be easily eliminated from the body.

How does all of this tie in with all-natural stevia and the man-made aspartame-containing sweeteners? We have learned from nutritionists and medical doctors that artificial sweeteners such as aspartame, which most people believe will help them to lose fat, actually cause fat gain by generating a false sense of hunger, which encourages overeating. With no compensating expenditure of energy, this results in excess fat storage. Researchers suggest that there may also be other factors that cause the brain to order the storage of fat when it becomes confused, and its normal processes are altered by the message input of these chemical sweeteners.

As early as 1986 the American Cancer Society documented the fact that persons using artificial sweeteners gain more fat than do the people who avoid them. Explains nutritionist Ann Louise Gittleman:

> The mere taste of such a concentrated sweetener appears to set an instinctual insulin mechanism into place even though aspartame contains zero calories. A six-year study of 80,000 women shows that the higher the artificial sweetener consumption, the more likely the women were to pack on the pounds.
>
> Aspartame, marketed under the Equal and NutraSweet brand names, also has been shown to suppress production of serotonin—the remarkable neurotransmitter that helps control food cravings. When serotonin levels plummet, those sugar and carb cravings skyrocket. And this increases the likelihood of bingeing and added pounds.
>
> Loading up on those diet drinks—sweetened by aspartame—

can rob you of valuable chromium, a mineral needed for proper blood sugar function. Having an insufficient amount of chromium results in poor blood sugar regulation, which can lead to insulin resistance and increased carb intolerance.[4]

Sandra Cabot, M.D., agrees. In a position paper she authored, she states emphatically that aspartame will cause fat gain, not fat loss. She writes:

> When you ingest the toxic chemical aspartame it is absorbed from the intestines and passes immediately to the liver where it is taken inside the liver via the liver filter. The liver then breaks down or metabolizes aspartame into its toxic components—phenylalanine, aspartic acid and methanol. This process requires a lot of energy from the liver which means there will be less energy remaining in the liver cells. This means the liver cells will have less energy for fat burning and metabolism, which will result in fat storing. Excess fat may build up inside the liver cells causing "fatty liver" and when this starts to occur it is extremely difficult to lose weight. In my vast experience any time that you overload the liver you will increase the tendency to gain weight easily.
>
> Aspartame also causes weight gain by other mechanisms. . . . [It] causes unstable blood sugar levels, which increases the appetite and causes cravings for sweets/sugar. Thus it is particularly toxic for those with diabetes or epilepsy. [It] causes fluid retention giving the body a puffy and bloated appearance. This makes people look fatter than they are and increases cellulite.[5]

To comprehend the magnitude of this condition of toxin overload, we must understand the importance of the liver. Scientists estimate that the liver performs 400 different functions, many of which are essential to health and to life itself. It is a living filter that cleanses the system of toxins, metabolizes proteins and carbohydrates, controls hormonal balance, enhances immune function, and synthesizes fibrinogen and other blood-clotting compounds that protect you from excess bleeding due to injury. The liver also directly affects your efforts to lose fat. The liver produces about a quart of bile each day and stores it in the gallbladder. When needed, bile is transported to the small intestine, where it emulsifies and absorbs fats. If not enough bile is produced, fat cannot be emulsified. This occurs when the liver lacks the required bile nutrients (cholesterol, bilirubin, lipids, lecithin, potassium, sodium, and chloride, carried in water, bile acids and pigments), is congested, or has clogged bile ducts.

"When your liver is sluggish, every organ in your body is affected, and your weight loss efforts are blocked," writes Ann Louise Gittleman.

> Blood vessels enlarge, and blood flow becomes restricted. A toxic liver is unable to break down the adrenal hormone aldosterone, which accumulates to retain sodium (and water) and suppresses potassium. This can raise your blood pressure. The liver fails to detoxify the components of estrogen (estrone and estradiol) for excretion, so symptoms of estrogen dominance arise. Unable to carry out its activities to control glucose, a toxic liver can lead to hypoglycemia, which can produce sugar cravings, weight gain, and Candida overgrowth. A toxic liver is unable to process toxins, enabling them to escape into your bloodstream and set off an immune response. With repeated assaults from escaped toxins, your immune system becomes overworked. Fluid accumulates, and you may develop one or more autoimmune diseases such as lupus or arthritis. A liver overloaded with pollutants and toxins cannot efficiently burn body fat, and thus will sabotage your weight loss efforts.[6]

As Dr. Cabot stated, the liver breaks down aspartame into its chemical components, which are toxic to the liver, thus exacerbating the complications and liver problems reviewed by Ann Louise Gittleman. This automatic response of the bodily process has motivated people to coin and promote the maxim: "If you want to get fat, aspartame is where it's at!"

ARTIFICIAL SWEETENERS AND SUGAR: AN INSIDIOUS DUO

Despite the vast amount of artificial sweetener in our current food supply, sugar consumption remains a devastating health problem. The reality is that the increased consumption of artificial sweeteners has not reduced our use of sugar. It has actually resulted in an increased consumption of sugar. Studies are beginning to suggest that artificial sweeteners actually increase the body's craving for sugar. During the 1700s the annual consumption of sugar was about one pound per person. By the end of the 1800s the yearly consumption had increased to about 16 pounds per person. Throughout the 1900s, with the advent of processed foods, consumption climbed rapidly. Today, following the introduction of artificial sweeteners into our foods and beverages, consumption of sugar in the United States averages an incredible 152 pounds per person per year!

You may think that this gluttony of sweets does not include you. However, if you check the labels on the cans, bottles, and boxes of processed foods on your shelves, you will discover the terrifying truth. Notice the total amounts of sugar, sucrose, dextrose, maltose, maltodextrin, corn syrup, fructose, caramel color, and similar hidden sweeteners used as ingredients.

While not yet backed by scientific research, myriad anecdotal reports indicate that stevia, in all of its forms, reduces the craving for sweets and fatty foods. You simply have less desire for them. Three or four such reports may be coincidental but dozens upon dozens add up to reality. Furthermore, stevia has this effect even though it has been scientifically proven to have zero calories and a glycemic index of zero. In stark contrast, Splenda, a popular sucralose product, has a glycemic index of 80; sugar has a glycemic index of 70; and fructose has a glycemic index of 20.

Scientific studies indicate that stevia, in its whole-leaf forms, nourishes the pancreas, the source of insulin regulation, and helps to correct and improve pancreatic function. In its refined, or extract (stevioside) forms, it has no effect upon the pancreas because it passes unchanged from the mouth to the anus and into the toilet. Thus, our tastebuds can enjoy stevia's wonderful sweetness with no harm resulting to any of the body's natural processes. However, if maltodextrin, dextrose, or another sweetener is blended with the stevioside, either as a filler or to achieve a certain taste profile, this noneffecting (bland) state is nullified and the pancreas and other bodily processes will suffer a reaction. It is of vital importance to read the label before purchasing or ingesting a product, including stevia products. The name of the product may be deceptive.

Another of stevia's many unique benefits (when unpolluted by other sweeteners), as reported by Linda Page, N.D., Ph.D., is that "stevia, a natural sugar substitute . . . significantly increases glucose tolerance and inhibits glucose absorption."[7] Stevia has no adverse effect upon pancreatic function, the liver, or the functioning of the body in the way it monitors and controls blood sugar levels. Nor does it cause a buildup of stevia metabolites within the tissues of the body or a stimulation to store fat.

However, researchers have written that in "aspartame poisoning" there is an accumulation of toxic poisons resulting in metabolic deficiencies that weaken the functioning of specific organs or even whole organ systems. Crash diets may worsen this problem. According to aspartame activist Georgia Conyers:

> In the case of aspartame and its breakdown components, the liver is largely unable to transform these poisons into an excretable form. When this happens, these toxins may infiltrate almost any area of the body that is weak and susceptible. . . . Most commonly, however, excess water and fat is retained by the body as a protective measure against the accumulated poisons. This is why a crash low-calorie diet is not recommended for weight loss. You may actually liberate the deadly poisons without assisting the body in their safe removal, further endangering vital organs and/or organ systems. Typically the nervous system is the most susceptible.[8]

Dennis Remington, M.D., and colleagues, in their book *How to Lower Your Fat Thermostat,* add this enlightening bit of knowledge, in answer to the question: Can artificial sweeteners be used instead of sugar?

> Although there are no calories in artificial sweeteners, they are not recommended for two reasons. First, artificial sweeteners seem to enhance the desire for sweets, and you may find it difficult to eat good, basic food without sweetening. Luckily, your tastes do change when you decrease the amount of sweets you eat, and food

such as cereals and grapefruit become very palatable. The second problem is that artificial sweeteners may also raise the setpoint.[9]

According to these experts, artificial sweeteners suppress serotonin, causing increased cravings for sweets and carbohydrates; raise your thermogenesis set point; and rob you of chromium, thus upsetting the insulin resistance mechanisms of your body, which causes your pancreas to increase your insulin production, in turn causing increased fat storage. Might this explain why more than 150 million Americans (about the same number of people advertised to be users of artificial sweeteners by the government and the manufacturers of NutraSweet and Equal) are storing too much fat and seem to be unable to lose it no matter what they do? Because they are continuously increasing their fat stores, they drink more diet beverages, switch to other diet plans, and eat more foods containing aspartame and other artificial sweeteners, exacerbating their problem. As Dr. David Williams, author of the health newsletter *Alternatives for the Health Conscious Individual,* writes: "Another side-effect of too much insulin is also not too well known. Excess insulin triggers a metabolic reaction that causes the body to store unusually large amounts of fat, particularly fat that has been ingested." He suggests "that a failure of the pancreas to properly control insulin may be one of the primary causes of obesity."

Dieting followed by overeating and then by dieting again may send a subconscious signal to the brain that a famine is about to occur and the body should therefore increase its fat storage. The brain is deceived into believing that we are constantly in or preparing for another famine, during which we must survive on stored fat. The input we give our brain by constantly eating beyond our satiation point overrules our conscious thought, or input from our mind, and causes our brain to raise our body's set point for fat storage. Simultaneously, our brain reduces our rate of thermogenesis and controlling set point, making it even more difficult to lose stored fat. Unfortunately, our conscious thoughts and decisions do not override the set point established, and adjusted by the brain as a means of survival, which is its fundamental responsibility. Besides, according to the visual input our brain receives from the outside world, many other people are also putting on and storing fat, so a famine really must be coming. The message to the brain is: "Everyone is preparing for a famine; store as much fat as possible."

When you "go on a diet," skip meals, or just eat less food, your brain believes that the famine has begun and lowers your body's set point, thus reducing your metabolism, or rate of burning available fuels, including stored fats. Reducing caloric intake appears to trigger a response within the body that slows the process of thermogenesis. Conversely, when you end the noneffective diet and resume eating a normal or even increased number of calories, your basic metabolic rate does not return to the prediet level. Dr. Remington suggests that "body fat is actually regulated by a control center in the brain," something he refers to as the weight-regulating mechanism, which actually "chooses the amount of body fat it considers ideal for your needs and then works tirelessly to defend that level," or set point. He says:

> This weight-regulating mechanism controls body weight in two important ways. First, it has a profound influence on the amount of food that you eat, dramatically increasing or decreasing your appetite as needed to maintain the setpoint weight. Second, it can actually trigger systems in the body to "waste" excess energy if you overeat, or to "conserve" energy if you eat too little. . . .
>
> Based on the nutritional needs of the body, you get a message to eat. While you have absolutely no control over the eating drive, you do have control over how you handle that drive. You decide when to eat, what to eat, and how much to eat. If you consistently eat less than your setpoint demands, the drive to eat may become so strong that the conscious, decision-making part of you will no longer be in control, causing you to eat quantities and kinds of food that will nudge the setpoint higher.[10]

At the same time, your body encourages you to decrease your activity level to conserve energy. This decrease in activity then affects your response to insulin, causing an increase in fat storage. Insulin is a hormone manufactured in the pancreas that is essential for getting glucose into the cell so it can be burned for energy (thermogenesis). Most obese people have too much insulin because their cells seem to be resistant to it. Their brain instructs their pancreas to produce more insulin to overcome the resistance. Exercise increases the ability of cells to respond to insulin and to produce energy and avoid fat storage.

INCINERATE YOUR FAT BY ACTIVATING YOUR BAT

It is also possible to reprogram your set point by making important lifestyle changes. The change in set point may not come quickly, so you must stay with the program. Begin by getting your body in shape, first exercising the large muscles used for walking and running for long time periods in a rhythmic manner. It is within these muscles that the greatest amounts of fat are burned. When the body gains muscle mass in the appropriate manner, it begins to believe that there is a need for greater sustained mobility. Since a more mobile person usually must be thin, the brain then orders the body to burn or waste even more fat. Eating the wrong type of foods will disrupt this process, as will eating behavior that kicks in the "famine is coming" mode. Says Dr. Remington:

> Exercise is a most critical factor in weight control. Inactivity is always detrimental. With a high activity level, the weight-regulating mechanism seems to sense the need for high mobility, the setpoint is lowered, and fat stores are "willingly" given up to produce a more streamlined, easier-to-move body.[11]

Dr. Remington teaches that both fats and carbohydrates are "burned" for energy in the muscles but that each has a separate metabolic pathway that depends on highly specialized enzymes for the process to take place. Exercise provides both the increased muscle and the specialized enzymes. The process is this: When an exercise period is begun, a molecule of fat is released from a fat cell and transported in the bloodstream to the muscle being stressed. "If there is sufficient muscle tissue that needs energy, and the muscle cell has fat-burning enzymes, the fat particle will move into the muscle and be burned," says Dr. Remington. "On the other hand, if a person has decreased muscle mass because of dieting, and has few enzymes for fat metabolism because of inactivity, the fat parti-cle will simply float around the system for a while, then return to the fat cell for storage."

In his book *Fat Management! The Thermogenic Factor,* Dr. Daniel Mowrey expands on the concepts of thermogenesis and the func-tion of brown adipose tissue (BAT) in burning white adipose tissue (WAT), or fat. He states that BAT is a special organ of the body whose sole purpose is to create heat by burning calories. "BAT is lo-cated between the shoulder blades, along the spinal column, atop the kidneys and in other discrete locations," he says. "Some experts believe that BAT may even occur intermixed with white adipose tis-sue." More recent research indicates that BAT is a special kind of in-sulating fat that is also found deep within the body. It surrounds the vital organs, including the kidneys, heart, and adrenal glands. It cushions the spinal column, the neck, and the major thoracic blood vessels. "When BAT thermogenesis is working, excess calo-ries are directed toward BAT where they are incinerated and dissi-pated as heat. When thermogenesis is not working, those extra calories are directed toward WAT where they are converted into stored fat molecules." Studies show, according to Dr. Mowrey, that "if the body loses its thermogenic capacity, obesity is certain to occur."

Ann Louise Gittleman writes that "BAT is dense in mitochondria [the power-producing structures in cells], giving the tissue its darker color. In mitochondria, nutrients are converted into a usable energy form through a set of reactions called cellular respiration. . . . BAT is high-energy fat. Its only job is to burn calories for heat. When properly activated, BAT can become your own fat-burning machine." She explains that "the omega-6 fatty acids stimulate your thyroid, thus raising your metabolism, and activate your brown adipose tis-sue (BAT) to burn fat rather than storing it in your white adipose tissue (WAT). . . . Thermogenic vitamins, minerals, herbs, and amino acids can help stimulate brown fat activity."[12]

Shivering produces small amounts of heat but BAT generates a more substantial amount. When we enter a chilly environment, we begin to shiver. This helps generate heat, but if the environment is too cold, this heat is not sufficient to keep us warm. Long-term exposure to cold requires heat to be generated metabolically through the process of BAT thermogenesis. We wear warm clothing to hold in that heat, preventing as much as possible from escaping into the atmosphere. When we were infants, we did not shiver. We had sufficient BAT to burn efficiently and help keep us warm when exposed to cooler temperatures.

The theory is that as we grow into maturity, we slowly lose this important tissue. Whether it shrinks or just atrophies, no one really knows. Researchers believe that it is a combination of genetic and behavioral factors. Behavior-wise it probably has to do with our mothers, who, listening to medical experts, obediently keep their homes warm and dressed their children warmly. (One of the foolish medical theories of years gone by was that if you become cold, you are more likely to catch a cold.) If you were like most children, you probably insisted that it was not that cold outside and that you were not cold when your mother demanded that you either wear your burdensome protective clothing or stay inside. When she looked out the window and saw that you had removed some of your layers of clothing, she chastised you, brought you back in the house, and perhaps even punished you. So you learned your lesson and began to overdress on your own and, according to the theory, began to lose your BAT.

I have personally observed a wonderful example of what Dr. Remington and Dr. Mowrey postulate in their books. My daughter Shannon, when she was twenty-five, spent two and a half months backpacking alone across the hinterlands of China, Tibet, and the Himalayas. She often hiked around 50 kilometers a day, carrying all of her possessions in a large backpack and eating the local food in the villages she visited. She was the only white, blond person some of the natives there had ever seen and she was often invited to join a local family for dinner. Because she speaks Mandarin Chinese, she could communicate with them. Some did not know that there were any languages except Chinese and Tibetan.

When Shannon returned home and told us of her experiences in the Himalayan Mountains, at about 18,000 feet altitude, and the glacier packs, her concerned mother asked, "Did you have enough warm clothing and coats? Did you have gloves?" Her polite response was, "Mother, I couldn't carry a heavy coat and gloves in my backpack. I had my light fleece sweater and a warm rain jacket. I was chilly, and sometimes very cold, but okay." She returned with a perfect feminine hourglass figure and not an ounce of fat. Clearly her set point had been lowered and her internal furnace had burned whatever excess fat she may have been carrying at the beginning of her trek.

My own BAT worked well until I was in my thirties. Perhaps I was blessed because we were financially poor when I was a child. I grew up in Phoenix, Arizona, where the winters were mild with morning winter temperatures only in the thirties and forties. On rare occasions, the temperature would dip into the high twenties. My parents couldn't afford to buy me two coats so I had only a light jacket and no other outerwear—which was sufficient. I was always reassuring Mother that I was not cold. And I wasn't cold, even though our early morning ballgame lasted from 7:30 until 9:00 A.M., when school started—and I played without a jacket.

By the time I entered high school, tightly fitting white T-shirts were the style for athletes. They showed off our rapidly developing biceps and triceps. The mornings were quite chilly but the afternoons were sufficiently warm. I decided that I'd rather be cold in the morning than have to carry a jacket after school, so I always left the jacket at home, until, of course, I won my varsity football and track letters in my sophomore year, to go along with my previously earned band letter. But my letterman's sweater was light, and I always wore it unbuttoned and sometimes just carried it slung over my shoulder. While I didn't know then that BAT existed, let alone that I possessed it, I suppose that being in the band as well as playing on the football team helped me to retain my BAT. Each winter day, the band members, bundled up in winter coats, practiced the marching routine for the next halftime show both before school and during morning band hour. However, since I would be playing football on Friday evenings, I would spend the entire early mornings in my gym shorts and T-shirt, so that I could use my breaks to jog or run on the track and fling my body, head first, into large and heavy blocking dummies. This was to prepare me, a ball carrier, for lowering my head and running into the huge linemen during the game. Good exercise for large-muscle development. Some of my friends continue to remind me that their funniest memory from high school was me playing a baritone horn solo, with band accompaniment, during a halftime show while wearing my full football uniform and pads with a band hat. (The coach wasn't happy that I wasn't in the locker room for his halftime motivational lecture, but he tolerated my experience.)

I kept up my practice of running during band halftime rehearsals during my first two years of college. I then spent the next two years taking a break from college and doing church service work in a very cold winter climate, however, so was given a warm overcoat by a family friend, to be worn with my scarf, earmuffs, and hat. Shivering was totally insufficient and so I wore the stuff. Homes were kept far too warm back then and apparently my BAT began to atrophy.

I spent the following two years in an equally cold climate, again attending college to finish my undergraduate studies. My parents had given me a three-quarter-length jacket, which I wore when it was really cold. When possible, I preferred the freedom of a long-sleeved flannel shirt. Constantly putting on a coat just to walk to another building for the next class, just to have to take it off again, was too much trouble for an Arizona boy, unless it was snowing. Besides, it felt good to be mildly chilly and it was only six blocks to the edge of campus from my off-campus room. Although I had an old car, I could not afford to buy gasoline so I didn't use it much.

I suspect that my brain-BAT signaling system was in a state of confusion. I got lots of sustained exercise in the cold, but my eating habits must have put my body into starvation mode, alerting it to create and store fat. My parents could afford to assist my educational experience with only $80 per month. I worked during the summers and part-time during the school year as a research assistant to one of my professors. The university paid $1 an hour but we students were allowed to work only nineteen hours a week. Money was in extremely short supply. I could afford to eat only one meal every third day in the university cafeteria. Since the friends with whom I ate that intermittent supper explained my plight to the food service ladies, my plate was always piled high with food. As a result, I gorged once every third day. When I had extra money, I would buy a box of dry cereal to keep in my room, an apple, or the largest candy bar I could find, preferably with lots of nuts, which I would eat for lunch or supper.

Family friends had moved to Provo, Utah, and their home was six blocks from Brigham Young University, the college I was attending. Because years before, I had helped their son during a time of difficulty, they invited me to live in a basement room—for free! So, although things worked out in terms of my educational endeavors, I suspect my fat-storing, fat-burning mechanism was in turmoil, not knowing whether to burn or store fat. After graduation in 1960 I returned to Phoenix. Following my marriage in 1963 I accepted a teaching position in Vernal, Utah, where it can be extremely cold in the winter. I relate this only to suggest that at that time my BAT was still functioning, providing necessary body heat.

In Vernal, my wife and I lived in a basement apartment. Early one winter morning (the first one there), I decided to help my landlord by shoveling the several inches of freshly fallen snow from his driveway. Wearing my Arizona short-sleeved shirt, I went outside to check the temperature. It felt chilly but not terribly cold, so in my short-sleeved shirt I commenced shoveling. About halfway through the job I called to my wife to suggest that it was so warm that spring must be coming. After completing the job, I noticed our landlord's outside thermometer. It was –10°F. In those days even with such temperatures, I wore only a suit coat to and from the classroom—but I did drive a car. However, in the years that followed, it became evident that my BAT had begun to atrophy and no longer functioned with such efficiency. Perhaps this happened because we moved back to warm Phoenix.

USE WISDOM TO BURN SUGARS AND FATS

If this current theory of fat storage–fat burning–fat waste is correct, coupled with the research concerning the extreme harm caused to the brain and bodily function by artificial sweeteners, I believe the most important criteria for fat loss and muscle maintenance are:

- Do not use artificial sweeteners, especially aspartame, whether in its generic form or consumer forms, including NutraSweet and Equal. Read labels and reject anything that contains an artificial sweetener.

- Adjust your set point downward via sustained, moderate, daily exercise, especially walking, jogging, swimming, hiking, bicycle riding, and jumping on a trampoline or minitramp. Remember also that the body has separate pathways for metabolizing fat and sugar. High-intensity activities cause the body to use the sugar pathway as its primary source of fuel. Heavy breathing is a sure sign that sugar is being burned as the primary source of energy. Moderate but sustained daily activity for longer periods of time encourages the release and burning of fat molecules and will, in time, bring about the results you desire.

- Eat a normal diet of healthy foods, primarily fruits, vegetables, beans, whole grains (with no sugar added), nuts and seeds, fish, and meat in moderation. As much as possible, eat raw, vine-ripened vegetables and fruits. Try buying whole wheat and whole oats in their natural forms and preparing your own highly nutritious cereals. Sweeten them with stevia.

- Do not dress too warmly during cold weather. Allow yourself to be moderately cool to encourage the possible regeneration of brown adipose tissue and to rev your metabolism for increased warming of the body and wasting of fat.

- Keep your cellular thermogenesis processes functioning. The thermogenesis occurring in each cell is minute, but when multiplied by billions of cells, the overall energy you use is significant. According to Dr. Remington, thermogenesis is a process involving sodium-potassium exchange. Therefore, it is essential that your body have a sufficient amount of these minerals. Obviously, too much sodium can cause water retention but too little sodium can hamper this important cellular function.

After all is said, written, and read, use wisdom in all things that you take into and put upon your body. There are numerous articles, books, and advertisements containing different people's theories on how to lose weight. But we are not all the same. What works for one person may not work for another. Many diets cause an initial loss of fat, but that fat is gained back once the diet is abandoned. If you want to lose fat and keep it off, you must examine your lifestyle and what you are willing to do for the rest of your life. Be reasonable, honest, and fair with yourself. It took time to put on the fat, and it will take time to get it off. Wisdom suggests that dangerous surgery should be the very last resort. Perhaps the very diet prescribed after such surgery, along with appropriate appetite suppressants, would be a better choice than surgery. Try the above suggestions for several months, replacing sugars and artificial sweeteners with your own preferred forms of stevia. Read labels, and remember to eliminate foods and drinks that are loaded with either sugar or artificial sweeteners. Move your body. Take the course less easily traveled. Use the stairs instead of the elevator. Walk as often as possible and burn stored energy.

7

Theoretical Science Uncovered

"He that walketh with wise men shall be wise:
but a companion of fools shall be destroyed."

—Proverbs 13:20

In 1992, in a report prepared for the FDA titled "Food Ingredient Safety Review: *Stevia Rebaudiana* Leaves," A. Douglas Kinghorn, Ph.D., professor of pharmacognosy at the College of Pharmacy, University of Illinois, Chicago, noted that "there have been well over 500 scientific articles" published about stevia and its safety.[1] And there have been dozens upon dozens published since 1992. In the preface to his latest scholarly work, *Stevia: The Genus Stevia*, released in 2002, Dr. Kinghorn reports that more than 1,000 studies and patents have been published about stevia.[2] We will review a few of these, as well as the pertinent conclusions reached by the scientists who performed the studies. To begin, let us review the negative studies upon which the FDA has been hanging its total "evidence" for rejecting stevia. It is important that we carefully examine these studies because those who want to discredit stevia continue to quote from them and to extrapolate potential consequences beyond the scope of the conclusions reached. They do this while totally ignoring the hundreds of studies that attest to the safety of stevia.

HYPOTHESIS: STEVIA IS A NATURAL CONTRACEPTIVE

In 1968, Gladys Planas, a chemist with the University of the Republic in Montevideo, Uruguay, and Joseph Kuc, a biochemist with Purdue University in Lafayette, Indiana, set out to prove that stevia is a natural contraceptive. When they began the study, they apparently knew just three things about the plant:

1. That it is "a Paraguayan weed" containing "a suprisingly sweet principle called stevioside."

2. That it was "prescribed" by Paraguayan physicians as a "hypoglycemic drug."

3. That the Paraguayan Motto Grosso Indian tribes used it as an oral contraceptive. Supposedly, the Motto Grosso women drank a "concoction in water from dry, powdered leaves and stems" every day.

The researchers state in their paper that they made no attempt to learn how the Motto Grosso women, or anyone else, used stevia for contraceptive purposes. Part of the reason could have been that no investigator has ever been able to locate any trace of the Motto Grosso. The whole story appears to be nothing more than a myth. The researchers therefore proceeded under the *assumption* that the tribe existed and that the tribal women drank a decoction made of dry stevia leaves and stems boiled in water. In fact, due to their total ignorance of the subject, they state: "Because of the lack of information concerning the amount of decoction that the Indians take, the calculations were made on the basis of our own experience acquired in northern Argentina with different weeds used as medicinals by the Indians." In other words, they prepared the stevia tea they used in their experiments according to the way a different tribe of natives, from a totally different culture, living in a different country, prepared teas using herbs other than stevia. In addition, after determing the amounts of "weed" and water theoretically used by an average woman weighing 60 kilograms (132 pounds) and converting the measurements for a female rat weighing an average of 0.250 kilogram (.55 pound), they *raised* the dosage to give the rats *eight times* what the women supposedly drank. They also prepared the tea by "boiling the dry, powdered weed in water for 10 minutes and filtering after cooling." That is, they boiled the entire plant, not just the leaves and stems.

The results the researchers obtained were that "fertility was reduced 57 to 79 percent in female rats drinking the decoction as compared to rats drinking water. A reduction of 50 to 57 percent in fertility was still evident 50 to 60 days after intake of the decoction had ceased." However, this statement does not reflect the true results, which were included in a chart in the report.

Specifically, the researchers carried out three experiments. In the first, they fed the stevia decoction to fourteen female rats for twelve days. As soon as each rat finished consuming her dose, which usually took about twenty minutes, her regular drinking water was returned to the cage. After the twelve days, the female rats were each put in a cage with a male rat to mate. During the six-day mating period, the researchers continued to give the females the stevia decoction. (They did not give the decoction to the males.) Thus, the females drank the strong decoction for a total of eighteen days. The researchers do not indicate that they observed any of the rats mating, only that they put the females with the males for six days.

The result of this first experiment was that three of the females given the decoction delivered 17 baby rats, or an average of 5.67 offspring per litter. In the control group of fourteen rats (not fed the decoction), eleven females gave birth to 78 rats for an average of 7.09 offspring per litter. Fifty to sixty days later, having been given only water to drink, the fourteen females in the test group were again placed with the males. This time, four of them produced 21 offspring for an average of 5.25 offspring per litter.

In the second experiment, the same procedures were followed. The results were that four of the fourteen test females produced 22 offspring, or 5.5 offspring per litter. In the control group, the fourteen females produced 91 offspring for an average of 6.5 per litter. Fifty to sixty days later, after drinking only water, six of the fourteen test females produced 32 offspring for an average of 5.3 per litter.

The third experiment was slightly different. Fourteen female rats that had never had the decoction were mated and produced 86 offspring for an average of 6.1 offspring per litter. A week after the offspring were weaned, or about twenty-eight days after giving birth, the females were started on the same treatment used in the first two experiments. After drinking the decoction for twelve days, they were mated with the same males that had fathered their first litters. Three of the females produced 21 offspring for an average of 7.0 offspring per litter. This was the same number of offspring per litter as produced by the control group in the first experiment.[3]

I Become the Surrogate Test "Rat"

To put the above experiments into perspective, I have calculated that an average person would need to drink a decoction made by steeping about nine tea bags of stevia in roughly one and a quarter cups of water to duplicate what was given to the rats. The taste of such a decoction would be so intensely sweet that no one would be able to tolerate drinking it. The usual recommendation is to use *one* tea bag to sweeten anywhere from two to six cups of water, depending on individual taste preferences.

Therefore, I have decided to try my own experiment, which I shall do right now, while I am writing this. Of course, I have already consumed three cups of a combination YerbaMaté Royale–pau d'arco tea this morning. As I have done for the past twenty years, I drink this blend every morning while I do my research and/or writing. It increases my mental alertness; significantly enhances my perception, thought processing, and memory; gives me physical energy and a wonderful sense of well-being; and eliminates my hayfever symptoms. The pau d'arco eliminates the pain of my old football injuries and reduces the inflammation in my nasal cavities caused by airborne allergies. So unlike the female rats in the study, I have consumed another liquid prior to the experiment.

I find a scale and weigh out how many tea bags I need. I find that I actually need *twelve* rather than nine. I allow 1.5 grams (.05 ounce) for the weight of the tea bag paper. I am most likely light in my estimated weight of the paper, so the weight of the stevia may be a few milligrams too light. I put 400 milliliters (13.5 fluid ounces) of water in a glass pot and bring it to the boiling point, estimating that 100 milliliters (3.4 fluid ounces) will boil away. I then add the twelve tea bags of stevia to the boiling water, and after ten minutes I remove the pot from the heat. As the decoction cools, I squeeze the tea bags with a spoon to filter out as much of the concentrated liquid as possible. I am left with 250 milliliters (8.5 fluid ounces) of highly concentrated stevia liquid to which I add 50 milliliters (1.7 fluid ounces) of clear water to get the prescribed 300 milliliters (10.2 fluid ounces) of decoction.

To my surprise, the decoction is not sweet. It is very bitter. It tastes so bad that in order to drink it, a woman or animal would have to be highly motivated or so very thirsty that she or it would be willing to drink anything. I debate with myself. Do I really want to do this? I know that this is far too great a concentration to drink at one time. Then, for the sake of true science, I begin to drink the foul-tasting substance. After all, I know that it won't kill me. Remember, I like stevia and have used stevia leaf daily for twenty years. I like the taste of stevia concentrate. In fact, I often squeeze a large amount of stevia concentrate directly out of the bottle into my mouth, add water, and use the blend as a mouthwash. When I have a sore throat, I swallow a whole mouthful of pure concentrate to stop the pain. Stevia concentrate has a strong but pleasant licorice flavor. But this stuff is bad! It takes a while but I am finally able to force it down.

Within two or three minutes I begin to belch stomach gas. I return to the computer to write. It is now twenty-five minutes since I drank the decoction and I feel nauseous and dizzy and find it difficult to think clearly due to the nausea. My stomach is growling and I am belching frequently.

It is now eighty minutes post drinking the decoction. The dizziness continues, as does the nausea. I have a slight pain in my stomach, heartburn, and a mild headache. I can't think clearly and it is difficult to type. I am really sick to my stomach. If my wife, whom I love dearly, were in town, there would be absolutely nothing that she—or any other female for that matter—could do to interest me in mating or doing anything of a romantic or intimate nature, be it physical or mental. Oh my, I know how those poor female rats felt. The females that did mate after ingesting this decoction were not normal. They must have been sex-crazed superrats! Or else the mating was not consensual. Poor defenseless things. I need to lie down for a while. I'm too sick to continue.

It is now four hours post experiment. I decide I cannot waste any more time lying down. I need to get back to writing this book. I have a deadline. When I sit up, the headache is significantly worse and persists. I drink a tall glass of water and eat some cereal, a banana, and whole-wheat toast to see if it will relieve my symptoms. No sweetener, please, I cannot bear to think of anything sweet. The nausea improves a little but the headache worsens. I rarely have even a mild headache. My progress in writing is very slow, as are my thought processes. I am making many errors, and am grateful I am using a computer and not a typewriter. I decide to drink more of my YerbaMaté Royale–pau d'arco tea blend because it also works to detoxify the body. I need to get this stuff out of my system. The belching has resumed and the mild stomach pain and slight pounding headache are continuing.

So that you may have a full understanding of the difference between the decoction I used in my experiment and the one consumed by the rats, I must give you the following information. Mine tasted much better and was more pure than what the rats got. Their drink was prepared by boiling the whole stevia plant, and was eight times stronger than mine—ugh! Mine was made using only leaves. When my Guarani Indian employees in Paraguay bring stevia into our factory from the plantation, it is the very best that has been produced that season. The plants are evaluated and the ones we use are carefully selected. When the plants are thoroughly dry, we hand-pick only the finest, best-quality leaves from each. We use no stems, no plant stalks, no blossoms, and no roots. We then cut and sift the leaves into tea bag size, and seal and store them in large plastic bags until they're needed. To make our stevia tea, we put the leaf particles into the hopper of the bagging machine, which seals them in tea bags; seal the tea bags in small plastic bags; and place the plastic bags in sales unit cartons.

In contrast, since the researchers considered stevia to be a weed, they apparently treated it like a weed. They do not indicate if the stevia they used was harvested wild or cultivated. Since it was for rats, however, I doubt that they kept it clean and uncontaminated. They also give no information regarding how the material was handled or if it could have been contaminated with other materials.

Observations and Conclusions

In my opinion, the study performed by Drs. Planas and Kuc was sloppy and poorly documented. It was based solely on assumptions and no facts. This was so from start to finish. The researchers wrote as if the Motto Grosso Indians still existed in Paraguay and yet did not bother to find out how, or if, they really used stevia as a contraceptive. They gave no positive identification of the plant material they used. Was it really stevia? Whatever it was, they considered it to be a weed, and they boiled the entire plant, not just the leaves. They gave no information regarding the plant being free of contaminants, nor did they mention if purity of sample was an issue. They never stated that they observed the test rats actually mating, only that the females were put with the males.

Based on my own experience, I don't believe that any female of any species that had to drink this decoction every day for eighteen days would have any desire to mate—even if the mate looked like Gary Grant, Pierce Brosnan, or Leonardo DiCaprio! She would be too sick to care. We all know the "Please, I have a headache" routine. Now I understand it. Anyone who accepts the Planas-Kuc study as scientific research needs to go back and retake high school Science 101. Surely, science—and the FDA—can do better than this!

Beyond My Own Experiment

Several laboratories have tried to duplicate the Planas-Kuc study but none has been successful. The female test animals become pregnant and produce normal-size litters of completely normal offspring. In an excellent review of the scientific literature concerning the safety of stevia, Dr. Kinghorn wrote, "Therefore, all scientific studies subsequent to the Planas and Kuc paper of 1968 have refuted these initial observations of an antifertility effect of *S. rebaudiana* leaves on male and female rats." In the same review, the doctor stated, "Recent inquiries in various regions of northeastern Paraguay, however, do not confirm the native use of *S. rebaudiana* extracts for contraceptive purposes."[4]

The footnote source that Dr. Kinghorn gives for this last statement is a report prepared for my Paraguayan company in 1991 by the National Institute of Technology and Standardization (NITS) in Asunción, Paraguay. The eight-page document was researched and written by Dr. Laura Fracchia, of the Instrumental Analysis Laboratory, and Dr. Miguel Gonzales Moreira, director of the Central Analysis Laboratory, and is addressed to me, James A. May. They were directed to prepare a complete review of the historical native use of stevia, including the initial and current scientific research and information on the herb. Their work was ordered by Dr. José Martino Vargas, general director of the NITS, of whom Colonel Luís Ramirez and I had made the request and whose fee for service I paid. Their complete review of the native use of stevia made no mention of the Motto Grosso Indians or of stevia ever having been used as a contraceptive. They did include a review of the Planas-Kuc study, which they indicated was refuted by two subsequent studies. Two of the subsequent researchers, following the Planas-Kuc study, said they believed that the contraceptive substance (if it existed at all) did not come from stevia leaves. The authenticated document, including a complete bibliography of the stevia research, was sent to me by Dr. Vargas along with a cover letter on August 27, 1991. Apparently Dr. Kinghorn obtained a copy from the Paraguayan government.

In a scientific paper published in 1985 in the journal *Economic and Medicinal Plant Research*, Dr. Kinghorn collaborated with Dr. D. D. Soejarto, also of the University of Illinois at Chicago, to prepare a lengthy and highly technical review of the scientific facts regarding stevia. This review included all the information available about the leaves and all the known medicinal, sweet, and other constituents therein, such as stevioside and rebaudioside A and their metabolites. Regarding the Planas-Kuc claims of antifertility, they wrote: "However, workers in several other laboratories have been unable to confirm this antifertility effect in rats. . . . Later inquiries made in several locations in northeastern Paraguay did not confirm the use of *S. rebaudiana* extracts for contraceptive purposes."[5] Dr. Soejarto had conducted a field study that included interviews with Paraguayan natives in several different regions where stevia grows naturally and is cultivated, including the Amambay region, where the plant originated. He could find no evidence that stevia had ever been used as a contraceptive either by the long-established Indians or by those who had recently come to the region.[6]

Numerous old reports and texts exist that list the various medicinal plants used by the natives of the region of South America now known as Paraguay. They contain no reference to the use of stevia, known by the natives as Ca á–Hê-é, for the purpose of contraception.[7,8,9,10,11,12,13] This suggests that the rumor of the Motto Grosso women using stevia as a natural contraceptive is totally false. However, reference is made to a different species of plant, *Stenosum variegatum,* being used by certain natives as a contraceptive.[14]

Now, a brief postscript about my experiment: Seven hours after drinking the decoction, I still have a headache, nausea, and general physical weakness requiring me to move more slowly than usual. My urine is bright yellow, indicating that my body is eliminating the high concentration of minerals from the stevia. My underarm perspiration has a strong stevia odor. I have to stop writing to take a shower and run some errands—albeit slowly.

It is now nine hours post stevia leaf decoction. I am still generally weak and have a headache and nausea but can function. I have appointments that I must keep even though I do not feel up to the tasks ahead.

Final Conclusion and Evaluation Concerning My Experiment

It took ten and a half hours for all of the effects of the stevia loading to pass and for me to feel normal again. Do not ever attempt to drink a stevia tea made with twelve tea bags and only one and a quarter cups of water. One tea bag to eight ounces of water is a very high concentration and is what is recommended for a seriously upset stomach or food poisoning—and it doesn't taste very good. On the other hand, one tea bag of stevia in a tall glass of tea or other beverage is both delightful and healthful.

There is wisdom in all things, and too much of a good thing can be harmful. Imagine trying to drink twelve tall glasses of water at one time. It could kill you. But that does not mean that water is harmful to your health. Only the abuse of it is harmful. It is the same with stevia. Always remember this: A little bit to a moderate amount of wisdom goes a long way.

HYPOTHESIS: NEITHER STEVIA NOR STEVIOSIDE POSSESSES CONTRACEPTIVE PROPERTIES

None of the data produced by other researchers in the 1970s supports the contraceptive claims of Drs. Planas and Kuc. Other scientists, however, wanted to make sure that no doubts remained. In 1981, N. Mori and colleagues fed pure stevioside to rats at the sweetness equivalent of 480 times a reasonable level of human intake. There was no evidence of a contraceptive effect and no effect on either fertility or the development of the offspring. The male rats were fed the stevioside for sixty days before mating and the females for fourteen days before mating and seven days after.[15] Note that this was not a stevia plant boiled in water but pure stevioside, which would have been 250 to 300 times sweeter than sugar.

In 1989, following their studies of the antifertility effects of stevia on rats, Dr. R. M. Oliveira Filho and colleagues stated that they could find no difference in the fertility of either male or female rats treated with stevia.[16]

An excellent study on both the safety of stevioside and its effect on reproduction was undertaken by scientists at the Primate Research Center of Chulalongkorn University in Bangkok, Thailand. These researchers presented a preliminary form of their findings at the 14th Conference of Science and Technology of Thailand in 1988, then published the complete results in the journal *Human Reproduction* in 1991. Having read the contradictory reports concerning the safety and contraceptive effects of stevioside, they had set out on their own road of discovery. I quote from their introduction to the published study:

> There were a few reports on toxicities of *Stevia rebaudiana* natural products in the literature. In an early report (Vignais et al., 1966) steviol was found to be a potent inhibitor of ATP synthetase in the isolated rat liver mitochondria. Further study (Wingard et

al., 1980) suggested the likelihood that stevioside would be converted into steviol in vivio and the converted substance would subsequently be absorbed through the gastrointestinal wall. Recently, metabolically activated steviol was found to exhibit mutagenic activity (Pezzuto et al., 1985) when tested against *Salmonella typhimurium*. As a result of a combination of these reports, stevioside may be expected to exhibit significant toxicity in humans. However, this expectation differs from many other studies. Oral administration of large quantities of stevia extracts, including large quantities of stevioside, revealed no acute or subacute toxic effect on mice (Akashi and Yokoyama, 1975) and rats (Lee et al., 1979; and Yamada et al., 1985). It was once reported (Inglett, 1979) that stevioside was non-toxic and passed unchanged through the human elimination channels. Moreover, no abnormalities attributable to consumed stevioside were observed in mating, fertility, or the development of fetuses (Mori et al., 1981). Neither did it promote urinary bladder carcinogensis in rats (Hagiwara et al., 1984). Due to the controversy of these reports, this work was carried out to investigate the effect of stevioside on growth and reproduction in hamsters.[17]

The study involved four groups of ten male and ten female hamsters, all one month old and weighing between 30 and 50 grams (1.1 and 1.8 ounces). Every day, the first group of hamsters was given 500 milligrams of stevioside for every kilogram of weight, the second group was given 1,000 milligrams of stevioside for every kilogram of weight, and the third group was given 2,500 milligrams of stevioside for every kilogram of weight. The fourth group served as the control group and received no stevioside.

Keep in mind that if a human adult weighing approximately 60 kilos, or 132 pounds, was given the dosage fed to the third group of hamsters, he or she would be taking about 150,000 milligrams, or 5 ounces, of stevioside. To comprehend the significance of this amount of pure stevioside (precisely 5.29 ounces), you should multiply the 5.29 ounces by 300 (stevioside is up to 300 times sweeter than sugar), which gives you 1,587.3 ounces. Divide this by 16 ounces and you find that 5.29 ounces of stevioside is the equivalent in sweetness of 99.2 pounds of sugar. For a human adult weighing 75 kilos, or 165 pounds, the sweetness equivalent would be 124 pounds of sugar. Ugh! That would surely kill you! But the stevioside did not harm the hamsters nor did it harm their off-spring. The point, however, is that no human being is going to ingest the stevioside equivalent of 99 to 124 pounds of sugar in one day—and then continue it every day!

You can imagine how awful this decoction must have tasted to the hamsters, which had to be force-fed. But the researchers state: "No abnormalities were found in growth and fertility in both sexes. All males mated females efficiently and successfully." They add, "Each female was mated and allowed to bear three litters during the period of the experiment. The duration of the pregnancy, number of fetuses, as well as the number of young delivered each time from females in the experimental groups were not significantly different from those in the control group." In other words, there was no significant difference in the average growth of the first generation of hamsters—no matter how much stevioside they were given.

The experiment was repeated with the next two generations of hamsters, with the animals "continuously receiving stevioside via drinking water until one month old and daily force-fed afterwards at the same doses as their parents [and they] showed normal growth and fertility. Histological examination of reproductive tissues from all three generations revealed no evidence of abnormality which could be linked to the effects of consuming stevioside."

Ray Sahelian, M.D., and Donna Gates also reviewed this study in their book *The Stevia Cookbook*. "As to the mating performance, all three generations performed the same, no matter which dose of stevioside they received," they concluded. "Their performance was equal to the controls. Microscopic examination of reproductive tissue samples from all of the groups, both male and female, of all of the generations, did not differ from the control group. The production of the sperm was normal, even in the males who received the highest dose of stevioside. In the females the ovaries of all of the animals were perfectly normal."[18]

Upon completion of the experiment, the researchers noted that the "results were quite astonishing. . . . We conclude that stevioside at a dose as high as 2.5 g/kg of body weight per day affects neither growth nor reproduction in hamsters. If this is true in other mammalian species including humans, this substance will be of great benefit to industry and medicine, and can be used more widely as a non-caloric sweetener in a variety of foods and drinks as already seen in Japan and Brazil."[19] Imagine that!

Now, let's look at the next research document the FDA uses to make stevia the "outlaw sweetener."

HYPOTHESIS: STEVIOL IS A CARCINOGENIC METABOLITE OF STEVIOSIDE

In 1979, researcher R. E. Wingard and his colleagues published their infamous study "Intestinal Degradation and Absorption of the Glycoside Sweeteners Stevioside and Rebaudioside A." This study was not in vivo—that is, it did not use live animals; it was totally in vitro—it used just laboratory test tubes. The purpose of the test was to determine if the stevioside metabolite called steviol, discovered by French chemists M. Bridel and R. Lavieille in 1931, would be absorbed through the intestine.

They faced a problem: How do you break down stevioside and rebaudioside A into basic metabolites? Bridel and Lavieille had accomplished the task in 1931 by enzymic hydrolysis using the hepato-pancreatic juice of the snail *Helix pomatia*. By this method they had discovered two aglycones, which they named isosteviol and steviol, and a unit of glucose.[20] Wingard and crew used a different method. They prepared a bacterial suspension (a specially created solution) by removing the contents from the cecum of a freshly sacrificed rat and adding them to a phosphate-dithiothreitol solution. They then gassed the suspension with an oxygen-free mixture of nitrogen and carbon dioxide, and passed the resulting substrate solution through Pyrex wool. The substrate solution was then divided into equal parts, and each part was gassed, tightly stoppered, and incubated at 37°C for periods of up to six days. Under these conditions of incubation 100 percent of the stevioside was converted into steviol in two days. However, it took six days for 100 percent of the rebaudioside A to be converted into steviol.

The researchers explain: "The objective was to simulate the occurrence of steviol in the intestinal tract following ingestion of the glycosides. Thus, the ethanolic dose, dispersed in aqueous hydroxypropyl cellulose, was injected intracecally into rats." That is, they injected this solution directly into the cecum of rats. Wingard and his associates extrapolated these data to humans and hypothesized that the human bowel *could* convert stevioside and rebaudioside A into steviol. In summation of this contrived research they wrote: "Stevioside and Rebaudioside A are degraded to the aglycone steviol by rat intestinal microflora in vitro. A similar degradation can be predicted to occur in man. Studies with steviol show the aglycone to be readily absorbed from the lower bowel of the rat. Analogous absorption from the human large bowel seems probable."[21]

Are they for real? I believe that this is an extraordinary stretch, and that this experiment provides absolutely no basis for their hypothesis that stevioside will be converted to steviol, by natural processes, within the human bowel. In fact, it has never been known to occur.

Do you have any of the stuff that they used to make the conversion in your intestines? I don't. Do you close both ends of your bowel with a stopper for two to six days? I won't. Perhaps this study should have been titled "From Test Tube to Homo Sapiens: The Hypothetical Stretch of the Century."

In their 1985 report, Drs. Kinghorn and Soejarto recognize that the data available on the metabolites of stevia are limited, but suggest that this study was done

> in spite of the fact that acute oral administration of large doses of stevioside and/or *Stevia rebaudiana* extracts and long-term studies with feeding either of these materials to laboratory animals have shown them to be virtually devoid of toxic effects. . . . Certain facts appeared to be presumed that may not be true in suggesting that humans would metabolize stevioside and/or rebaudioside A to steviol, which would then be absorbed, following oral administration. Stevioside and rebaudioside A were metabolized in the Wingard studies to steviol in vitro by rat cecal flora. Humans do not have a cecum, and it may be anticipated that the microbial flora of the human intestinal tract contains different microorganisms than does the rat cecum. Thus, it remains to be shown that the microbial flora of other species, or that of humans, will metabolize the stevia sweet

principles in a manner analogous to that described by Wingard and co-workers (1980).[22]

In his 1992 report, prepared for the Herb Research Foundation as part of its FDA petition, Dr. Kinghorn was a bit more expressive regarding Dr. Wingard's extrapolation. "Wingard and co-workers (1980) extrapolated their rat data to the human situation, and have suggested that the human bowel could convert over 0.4 g rebaudioside A to steviol each hour," he wrote. "However, this calculation may be somewhat presumptuous because humans do not have a functional cecum and therefore contain different intestinal tract microbial flora than the rat."[23]

Rats are scavengers. They often live in and devour all kinds of garbage. They will eat nearly any kind of plant or other animal, dead or alive—even other rats. They will gnaw on walls, furniture, lead pipes, and the insulation covering electrical wiring. Their digestive systems were designed to process such materials. Dr. Daniel Mowrey was correct when he said, "Humans are different from rats."[24]

In an exhaustive review of the scientific literature on this subject for the United Medical and Dental Schools at Guy's Hospital in London, Keith Phillips wrote:

No evidence was available in the 1970s to suggest that steviol or isosteviol are produced from stevia in humans. The only enzyme systems known to degrade stevioside to steviol and glucose had been demonstrated in:

- heptic pancreatic juice of the vineyard snail *Helix pomatia;*
- gastric juice of the marine snail *Megalobalimus paramaguensis;*
- pectinase
- crude hesperininase

No enzyme in the human digestive system was known to have a similar action. The report by Vignais et al. that steviol and isosteviol inhibit oxidative phosphorylation in vitro would not therefore have been considered significant, especially with the total lack of evidence for any toxic effect from the acute and sub-acute feeding data.[25]

With all these facts before you, where would you place the results suggested in the Wingard study? Would you call it science? Did they establish any facts as they relate to living human beings? Did they discover sufficient evidence to move their predetermined result to the realm of theory? Or must this study remain in the realm of hypothesis—meaning that no evidence was discovered indicating that their findings might also apply to the intestinal tract of a human? I believe the facts are clear: This study was manipulated and its stated results contrived. As it pertains to human beings, I believe it is without merit.

Does this not beg questions such as: What is the true motivation behind these negative studies? Why are such farfetched extrapolations being made in order to postulate a negative possibility? Who is funding this research, designed and contrived to darken the bright aura that surrounds stevia? Who stands to lose if stevia is accepted as the most desirable sweetener in the future? What will happen, and to whom, should the extraordinary sweetening and healing benefits of stevia become known to the people of the world? What if diabetics and hypoglycemics become aware that stevia and stevioside can help their conditions? What if people learn that one of the most effective first-aid products on earth is stevia leaves in a water-based concentrate? What if people find that this same stevia concentrate might help cure skin cancer? Who stands to gain? Who stands to lose?

But to be fair, we must continue our quest to discover the true scientific facts as they relate to stevia and stevioside. In 1984, John M. Pezzuto and his colleagues were able to create steviol in a relatively complex process by treating stevioside with sodium periodate and sodium hydroxide. They then used this laboratory-created steviol to treat a strain of bacterium, *Salmonella typhimurium* TM677, in a test commonly used to determine toxicity. When they treated the bacteria only with steviol, nothing happened. They found that to obtain the toxicity they were looking for, they had to pretreat the bacteria with a special chemical obtained from the livers of rats, which also had to be chemically pretreated.

By using a metabolic activating system—which they had to prepare in the laboratory—they were able to induce a mutagenic effect upon the bacteria. They added the bacteria to the test substance, which they had dissolved in dimethyl sulfoxide and slowly rotated at 37°C for two hours. They then quenched the reaction by adding phosphate-buffered saline. They recovered the bacteria by centrifugation, resuspended it, and allowed it a growth period of thirty-six to forty hours at 37°C. Following this procedure they noted mutagenic activity upon the bacteria. "It is likely that covalent interaction with bacterial DNA occurs," they suggest. Notice that they do not say the DNA of the bacteria was altered, or how it could have been altered. They merely postulate that it is likely it was altered.

This study is used by the opponents of stevia to suggest that steviol is mutagenic and, therefore, may be harmful to humans. However, that is not at all what the study demonstrated. According to the conclusions reached by the researchers, "When evaluated at steviol concentrations as high as 10 mg/ml in the absence of the S-9 fraction, however, no significant activity was detected."[26] In the study the researchers state:

Consistent with reports in the literature, we have found that stevioside is not mutagenic as judged by the utilization of *Salmonella typhimurium* Strain TM677, either in the presence or in the absence of a metabolic activating system. Similar negative results were obtained with several structurally related sweet-tasting glycosides. However, steviol, the aglycone of stevioside, was found to be highly mutagenic when evaluated in the presence of a 9000 x g supernatant fraction derived from the livers of Aroclor 1254-pretreated rats. Expression of mutagenic activity was dependant on both pretreatment of the rats with Aroclor 1254 and addition of NADPH; unmetabolized steviol was not active. The structurally related isosteviol was not active, regardless of the metabolic activation. . . . Finally, it should be emphasized that no reports have thus far appeared indicating that adverse effects have resulted from human use of stevia products. Other substances found in the diet are known to mediate mutagenic responses with no apparent impact on health. Based on the results described herein, to potentuate the mutagenic effect, it would first be necessary to produce the aglycone of stevioside and then metabolically activate this species.[27]

In their concluding statements, they write: "Thus, it seems unlikely that stevioside would be degraded to steviol when subjected to typical methods of cooking, storing or processing." Not only is it unlikely, it is virtually impossible!

In view of all of the conclusions reached by the scientists, their final statement is both perplexing and mystifying. "Nonetheless, complete metabolic conversion of stevioside to an active mutagenic species by human enzymic systems involved in the biotransformation of endogenous substrates or xenobiotics is possible," they write. "It therefore appears that adequate information is currently not available to condone the widespread human consumption of stevioside. Additional studies relevant to safety assessment are required."[28]

If this transformation is possible, why did they not explain just how it is possible? Better yet, why did they not utilize this possible method of transformation in their research? If they do not know how to achieve the transformation, what makes them think that it is possible, especially in the human intestinal tract? Finally, what motivated them even to make such a statement when it is totally undocumented and negated by their own study? It's a mystery.

Are we too bold to suggest that the display of systematic scientific piety regarding manipulated research in the interest of private greed or ambition is the epitome of academic shortsightedness? In the end, true science will prevail, and all the shadowy figures will silently fade into the darkness of oblivion.

Philippe Shubik, M.D., of Green Gollege, University of Oxford, reviewed the Pezzuto study in a report titled "Toxicological Review of *Stevia Rebaudiana*":

> Studies by Pezzuto et al. demonstrating that a metabolite of the aglycone steviol can induce forward mutations in *Salmonella Typhimurium* TM677 is clearly of academic interest. It had been suggested by these authors that this might indicate that stevioside could pose a carcinogenic hazard. This is a somewhat tenuous proposal that would require the hydrolysis of stevioside to steviol in the human [intestines] and subsequent specific metabolic conversion of steviol to the metabolite inducing this mutation. It must be noted that both stevia and the several glycoside constituents as well as the aglucone steviol are quite negative in a series of Salmonella assays designed to determine reverse mutations; little credence is

given to overall toxicological evaluations to mutagenicity findings in the presence of a negative chronic toxicity study. In addition, the use of studies with TM677 demonstrating forward mutations, although of considerable academic interest, has not found favor with those engaged in using these tests as screening procedures for possible carcinogenesis.[29]

With that in mind, now read the statement neatly tucked away in the middle of the Pezzuto document: "Although unlikely, it was of concern that a small quantity of a chemical contaminant might have copurified with the steviol and elicited the mutagenic/bactericidal response."[30] How in the world do you copurify a substance with a chemical contaminant?

Forgive me. I cannot resist the temptation. The comparison must be drawn. The FDA considers herbal products and other nutritional supplements to be adulterated when their manufacturers provide truthful information to consumers concerning their beneficial uses. Here, the scientists consider that when a toxic contaminant has been added to their test solution, the solution has been "copurified." Apparently the FDA is willing to accept this anomaly because it uses this study to claim that stevia may cause harm to humans. It figures.

ONE FINAL BUT HIGHLY IMPORTANT STUDY

"Assessment of the Carcinogenicity of Stevioside in F344 Rats" is the title of an article published in the June 1997 issue of *Food and Chemical Toxicology*. This research project was performed by Dr. K. Toyoda and his colleagues at the Division of Pathology of the National Institute of Health Sciences in Tokyo, Japan. In their conclusion, the researchers say that the information concerning steviol given in other studies, including the ones we discussed in this chapter, "with regard to mutagenic potential is intriguing, given the lack of carcinogenicity found in the present study." Take note of their use of the word *intriguing*. This is scientific verbiage used in place of the statement, "There are basic errors in the study. Therefore the conclusions extrapolated are in error." The researchers mention that they did find steviol in the contents of the large intestines of rats treated with stevioside in one of their previous but unpublished studies, "as in the present [published] carcinogenic study."

Their previous study is also extremely intriguing, given that 10 percent of the diet fed to the test rats consisted of stevioside. That's an incredibly huge amount! If you ate 3 pounds, or 48 ounces, of food per day, you would be consuming 4.8 ounces of stevioside sprinkled on 43.2 ounces of food. Since stevioside is up to 300 times sweeter than sugar, 4.8 ounces of stevioside is equivalent in sweetness to 1,440 ounces, or 90 pounds, of sugar. Can you imagine having to eat 90 pounds of sugar sprinkled on 43.2 ounces of food every day?

The rats in the previous, unpublished study were sacrificed after two days, one week, two weeks, and six weeks. The contents of their large intestines were collected in a 50 percent methanol solution, and quantitative analysis revealed steviol in this material. The greatest amount of steviol, however, was in the rats killed after only two days. Each succeeding group had a smaller amount of steviol in its intestinal contents. The smallest amount, which was so tiny it was almost nonexistent, was in the rats examined after six weeks. The two-day group had 5.1 milligrams per rat, the one-week group 2.8 milligrams per rat, the two-week group 2.8 milligrams, and the six-week group 1.1 milligram.

The fact of greatest importance here is not whether the stevioside was converted into steviol in the cecums of these rats or after retrieval through the use of the methanol solution but that within seven days the rats were either eliminating it with astounding efficiency or not converting as much. The more stevioside they ate, the more proficient they became at producing less or at eliminating converted steviol in their waste. So what is the problem?

The other fascinating observation to be made about this study and the others is that when rats were injected with stevioside that had been metabolically activated with toxic chemicals and converted into steviol in the laboratory, they seemingly were unable to eliminate it. When they ingested the stevioside naturally, as part of their diet, they were very efficient at eliminating the steviol and were totally unharmed by it. Note that neither mutagenicity nor carcinegenicity was found in any of the rats in these two experiments. "Therefore the conclusion that stevioside exerts no carcinogenic activity in F344 rats when administered continuously in the diet at concentrations of 2.5 or 5 percent for up to 104 wk, presumably also means that any mutagenicity exerted by steviol is not of significance for neoplasia under these circumstances," the researchers concluded.[31] So, as we have observed in these two studies, even though some stevioside was apparently converted into steviol in the large intestines of the rats, it did no harm. Furthermore, the rats' bodies became extremely efficient at eliminating it.

Ray Sahelian provides an excellent review of this published study, and certain specifics of the findings of the scientists:

> For a period of 104 weeks (2 years), three groups of lab rats—fifty male and fifty female—were tested. One group received stevioside in a concentration that constituted 2.5 percent of their daily diets; the second group received a concentration that constituted 5 percent of their daily diets. The third group, which served as control, received no stevioside. At the end of the study, all of the surviving rats were euthanized. The rats who received the stevioside weighed less than those in the control group. Considering stevioside has no calories, this makes sense. When the organs and tissues of the rats were examined under a microscope, there was almost no difference between those who were given stevia and those who were not. One interesting difference, however, was that the females who took the stevioside had a decreased incidence of breast tumors, while the males displayed a lesser incidence of kidney damage.[32]

Enough said?

I am fascinated by the reduced incidence of breast tumors in the female rats. During the last twenty years, numerous women have called to tell me about what they considered to be a miraculous experience. They had read about a recipe that I learned from the Guarani Indians of Paraguay. When they drank the special home-prepared tea—made of a combination of pau d'arco, yerba maté, and stevia leaf—their breast tumors disappeared, often in only two weeks, and their physicians informed them that no surgery was necessary. I had no idea that stevia might have been involved in their healing process until I read this study. The healing potential of some herbs is absolutely incredible.

God created plants and herbs for certain needs, and man must learn to use them with skill and wisdom, for the purposes for which they exist. Some were created for food for man and animals, some for medicines, some for clothing, some for houses, some to provide nourishment for other plants. Some were made to please the eye and to gladden the heart. Some were created to delight the mouth and the nose, others to strengthen and invigorate the body and to enliven the soul of man. There is wisdom in all things. There is wisdom in herbs. Thank God for the wonder of herbs.

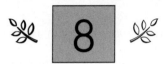

Special Reports: Europe and Canada

"Patent a synthetic sweetener, do some toxicity studies in animals that show it to be safe, send the results to the FDA for their stamp of approval, and you're instantly a billionaire. It's that easy. Actually, even if the artificial sweetener is suspected of causing cancer in animals, and you happen to have a great lobbying team, you can still make your billions. But if you happen to want to sell a natural product as a sweetener that has been used for centuries and has not been shown to cause toxicity in animals and humans, good luck."
—Ray Sahelian, M.D., and Donna Gates,
The Stevia Cookbook: Cooking with Nature's Calorie-Free Sweetener (Avery, 1999)

Much misinformation has been disseminated by writers concerning the refusal of the European Commission to approve the use of stevia in Europe. While the statements made by the commission are factual, unless you understand the background of the ruling and the course of events that led to it, you will not comprehend the reasons behind it. I was there as the complex drama began to unfold. I played a role in attempting to provide the stevia safety studies to the Belgium Health Ministry. The ministry wanted access to the scientific studies, but their own rules would not allow them to receive the materials from anyone other than the petitioner. It was a lesson in futility for the Belgium health authorities, the citizens of Europe, and me. When denied the very data required, it is impossible to make an informed and correct decision.

THE EUROPEAN COMMISSION

In October 1998 I went to Europe to work with the executives of companies who wanted to market stevia. Our experience in Brussels, Belgium, was unique and explains the position of the European Commission.

We had shipped a half-ton of ground stevia leaf to Rudi De Kerpel in advance of my arrival. His people had designed their own label and had packaged the product, which we were to introduce in a specially designed exhibit at a large European food trade show. The exhibit and label were designed around the theme of an ancient Guarani Indian village. It was a very popular display. Free samples of the product were given to eager and grateful attendees. We were interviewed by many local officials, writers for magazines, and the press. Our pictures and the story of stevia became a featured article in the major newspaper. We received calls from executives of companies in several European countries and the Middle East, who wanted to market our stevia.

At a dinner gathering Rudi and his attorney-partner, Serge Grysole, informed me of the current situation regarding stevia in Europe. A professor at the university had been growing stevia in a greenhouse for research purposes. At the conclusion of his project he did not know what to do with his 80,000 healthy stevia plants. Learning of the professor's dilemma, Rudi had called him with a solution. Since Rudi also owned a few plant nurseries and was the buyer for several others, he would offer them for sale to the general public. They were all sold within two weekends.

The Belgium equivalent of the FDA charged Rudi with selling an unapproved food. No one had yet obtained government approval to market stevia, although we had been shipping smaller amounts of the herb to companies and individuals in several European countries for years. Stevia was, however, under review by the authorities. The case went to court, where the judge ruled that stevia, as a plant, did not come under the jurisdiction of the agency. Selling stevia plants did not violate the law. Apparently this judge understood that selling stevia leaves was no different from selling lettuce, carrots, or tomatoes. Stevia is simply a vegetable, which consumers have the right to purchase and eat.

Since there was no real difference between marketing living stevia plants from which people could pick and eat the leaves and selling ground stevia leaves, Rudi introduced the product at the food trade show. On October 16, 1998, we met with Raoul Verschueren, assistant to the minister of health in Brussels. Our purpose was to inform him of our plans to market the various forms of stevia in Belgium. We anticipated that with the recent court decision, our timing would be perfect and that there would be no objection.

Verschueren informed us that the professor had submitted a request to the Belgium authorities to approve stevia as a "novel food." If approved in Belgium, then due to the recent European trade agreement, it would automatically be approved throughout Europe. However, if the Belgium authorities denied the petition, all the European nations must do the same. Having been aware of Rudi's victory in the Belgium court, the professor had seized the opportunity for economic reward. He had submitted the request the previous February, under the Novel Foods and Novel Foods Ingredients Act, and had submitted an updated, final version, with an addendum, on September 21, 1998.

We asked how the hearings were proceeding. "Not good for stevia," Verschueren replied. "We have asked the professor for scientific studies that show stevia is safe for human consumption. He said that he is the professor, and that we need no other studies than his own. He said, 'I am the authority here, and you need no proof except my word. I say stevia is safe and that is all you need to know.' He adamantly refuses to submit other studies." Verschueren then added that he felt the commission would deny the petition for lack of relevant scientific data. I told him that I had those very studies with me, and asked permission to submit them to the committee myself. He said that the rules did not permit anyone but the petitioner to submit evidence. He suggested that we give the studies to the professor for submission. We agreed. I got the feeling that he favored the approval of stevia but felt that without good science to back it up, the commission would deny the approval.

Rudi, using his cell phone, called the professor and told him that I was in Belgium, had scientific studies with me that had been performed by scientists around the world, and offered them to him. They would prove that stevia is completely safe. I was standing next to Rudi and could hear the professor shouting, "Who is Jim May? I do not know Jim May. I am the authority on stevia. No one knows more about stevia than I do. They must accept my studies! I need no help from you!" He slammed down his phone in Rudi's ear. I believe there is no ignorance like arrogance. We correctly feared that the future of stevia in Europe was in peril.

Not being allowed to provide the very scientific studies that would prove the safety of stevia, we could only wait and hope that the professor would come to his senses. Apparently he didn't. The committee ruled against stevia because of the lack of relevant studies proving its safety—not because they did not exist, but because they had not been submitted to them. The European Commission had no choice but to follow suit. A few of the comments of the commission, as contained in their official decision, are revealing:

> . . . and no analytical data have been supplied. No inherent toxic components are described but again no analytical evidence for their absence has been supplied. No microbiological specification has been supplied.
>
> The fresh leaves are used in very small amounts and therefore most unlikely to replace other vegetable foods to any significant extent. The dry powder is intended to replace some of the sucrose in drinks, jams and sweets to reduce the caloric intake. It may be used by diabetics and overweight individuals. No relevant studies have been submitted to show the physiological and pharmacological effects of this substitution on diabetic or obese individuals. No studies have been submitted showing the effect of the addition of the powdered material on the bioavailability of macro and microconstituents of the normal diet.[1]

The conclusion of the official decision added:

> The information submitted on the plant products was insufficient with regard to the specification and standardisation of the

commercial products and contains no safety studies. There are no satisfactory data to support the safe use of these products as ingredients of food or as a sucrose substitute for diabetics and obese individuals. The only toxicological data submitted are essentially concerned with the stevioside component of the plant product. No appropriate data were presented to enable the safety of the commercial plant product to be evaluated.[2]

The commission issued another opinion on the same date. It concerned stevia used as a sweetener, and was requested by a company in Italy. The request was apparently the result of an agreement made between the company and a chemist-industrialist in Paraguay who had developed a method of extracting the sweet glycosides from stevia leaves using a solvent made of orange juice and sugar cane juice. This new extraction method was a novel idea and resulted in a stevioside that is delicious. I own the rights to market this product in North America, and in my discussions with the industrialist, I had learned that the European rights were held by an Italian company. The industrialist's Paraguayan factory was built and ready for operation. I toured his factory, his sugar cane fields and extraction facilities, and his laboratory.

The Paraguayan industrialist had three major obstacles. The first problem was that he had produced his stevioside only in his laboratory, never in commercial production. He had invested $10 million in American money in the project, borrowed from a Brazilian bank. Second, there was no market for his product in Europe until approval was granted. And third, although I could (as of 1995) market the product in the United States, his extraction method was far too costly, resulting in a price that put him totally out of the competitive race. Chinese industrialists, supported by government subsidies, won the race for a competitively priced product.

The 1999 opinion rendered by the European Commission indicated that the committee had first reviewed stevioside as a high-intensity sweetener in 1985, and then again in 1989. Stevioside was denied as a sweetener both times. Why? A careful reading of the statement issued by the committee makes the reason painfully obvious. Whoever prepared the review of the data for the commit-

tee, as well as for the European Commission, did not want stevioside to be approved, and stacked the deck against it. The only other
possibility is that they did not understand what they read or did
not read the studies carefully. The studies used were the very same
ones the FDA used when denying stevia.

The studies referred to in the opinion issued by the Scientific
Committee on Food are the one by Drs. Kuc and Planas that claims
stevia acts as a contraceptive (we have analyzed this study and
found it to be without merit); the one by Dr. Wingard and colleagues that erroneously postulates stevioside to be mutenagenic
via the production of the metabolite steviol; and the Pezzuto study
of metabolically activated steviol. Whoever prepared the data for
the committee made questionable statements regarding the conclusions of the scientists. In one place the writer states that Wingard
"concluded that degradation of stevioside *may* occur in man." We
know that Wingard postulated that degradation of stevioside might
occur in man but it has never been known to occur. It is, in fact,
impossible because of the difference between the contents of the rat
cecal microflora and that of the human cecumless intestinal tract.
In the conclusion of the opinion, the writer boldly—but inaccu-
rately—states, "Futhermore, steviol, one of the metabolites of stevioside, that is produced by the human microflora is genotoxic and
induces developmental toxicity."

The opinion also reports that the studies state that stevioside results in changes in the male reproductive system, which we have
also found to be unreliable, and which are totally refuted by later
studies where the male rats were allowed to copulate normally with
females. The opinion adds, "Thus, it can be concluded that steviol,
but not stevioside, seems to induce developmental toxicity in high
doses."[3] It closes with this:

> In the safety assessment of the specific stevioside preparation for
> which approval is sought, several questions of concern were raised
> by the Committee regarding the specifications of the extracts that
> had been tested, questionable chronic toxicity and carcinogenicity
> studies, and possible effects of the male reproductive system that
> could affect fertility. Furthermore, steviol, one metabolite of stevio-

side, that is produced by the human microflora is genotoxic and induces developmental toxicity. The Committee is not satisfied with the submitted documentation and has concern about possible toxicity. Areas that need further studies are stated in the above opinion. The Committee reiterates its earlier opinion that the substance is not acceptable as a sweetener on the presently available data.[4]

When an investigating committee or ruling commission is not given accurate and truthful information, it is difficult to expect appropriate decisions to be rendered. No one need fear using stevia or stevioside as the food if it is as a result of the decision made by the European Commission. I believe that whoever prepared the report either lied to the committee or simply could not understand the science involved.

THE CANADIAN GOVERNMENT

Two agencies of the Canadian government are working to develop new varieties of the stevia plant and new methods for extracting the steviosides and rebaudiosides from their leaves. I have met with officials and scientists from these organizations and toured their agricultural projects and extraction facilities. When I asked an official of the National Research Council of Canada about stevioside not being allowed in his country, he replied, "When we are ready and present our data, our products will be approved by the government." The researchers have not yet proven their methodology nor its cost-effectiveness.

Whole-leaf stevia products and stevia extract products are permitted in the Canadian market. My company sells these products to many stores and distributors. In fact, during the year 2000, the Canadian government featured the stevia, stevioside extract, and SteviaPlus products of Wisdom Herbs at an international trade show, and samples of single-serving packets of SteviaPlus were distributed to the attendees at the government's exhibit. They wanted industrialists from around the world to realize the potential of producing consumer products with stevia.

* * *

As stated at the beginning of this chapter, when the individuals, committee, or organization that is required to make a decision is denied the factual information it needs to make the decision, it cannot make a correct judgment. Further, we want desperately to believe that the men and women in governmental positions of authority who make decisions concerning our lives and our health and well-being have our best good in mind. While most of them do, I don't believe that all do. Unfortunately, all these people are human, and the desire for wealth, power, and fame all too often clouds the mind and heart, adversely affecting good judgment and altruism.

Money breeds power, and power is often the predecessor of corruption. Power corrupted has the ability to sustain its own flow of money and influence at all levels of community, business, and government. The past decade has witnessed horrific examples of individuals, corrupted by corporate and governmental power and filled with personal greed, who forgot they were appointed or elected to be servants of the people and to make life better for all.

Many nations around the world look to our own FDA as the standard for determining the safety of foods and drugs, and thus the health and well-being of their citizens. Has the FDA lived up to this trust? I believe that regardless of how good the structural foundation is—whether the entity is a governmental organization, a private agency, a corporation, or a family—occasionally a rotten apple may rise to the top, gain power, and act in self-interest rather than for the good of the whole. It is a true maxim that one rotten apple, if not removed in time, will corrupt many of those nearby, and the stench may adversely affect the entire barrel.

I suggest that just as in individuals, the strength of the FDA is also its weakness. The FDA looks at science, as well it should. That is its strength. It is also its inherent weakness. FDA commissioners are generally selected from among the administrators in the world of pharmaceuticals and medicine. Its scientific advisors are often selected from the very corporations these commissioners once governed or with which they competed. Their knowledge base is confined to the world of their own training and paradigm. Once their term of service has expired, these individuals return to the world of creating, obtaining approval for, and dispensing drugs, medicines, medical devices, and medical services. Thus, their paradigm is narrow, and the pressures exerted upon them by the industry of their captivity are enormous.

It is well understood that creating a substance the FDA will approve as a sweetener is the golden pathway to billions of dollars in annual revenue. What are men and women willing to do to obtain such revenue? Perhaps the story of aspartame will help us to understand the answer to this query and to better comprehend the old maxim, "Let the buyer beware."

Aspartame: The Most-Studied Product in History?

"Aspartame is potentially dangerous and may produce a wide variety of physical and mental symptoms, most of which now go unrecognized or are misinterpreted as serious illnesses. . . . In fact, I believe that products containing aspartame are capable of producing, and reproducing, a wide spectrum of frightening symptoms, including severe headaches, convulsions, memory loss, and diarrhea—to name just a few."

—H. J. Roberts, M.D., *Aspartane (NutraSweet): Is It Safe?* (The Charles Press, 1990)

Aspartame, known better by its consumer trademark names *NutraSweet, Equal,* and *Spoonful,* is now consumed on a daily basis and often in very large amounts, by more than 150 million people in the United States. It is used as a sweetener in thousands of products including vitamins, medicines, and treats designed for children. H. J. Roberts, M.D., acknowledged as the world's leading authority on aspartame, estimates that it is currently used in more than 9,000 products. It is added daily to hot coffee, hot chocolate, and other beverages by tens of millions of people. Parents give it freely to their children in soft drinks and desserts. But do you really understand what this product is, or the effect it has had on people since its introduction as a sweetener? In this chapter, we will discuss the true scientific and consumer "anecdotal" facts concerning this substance.

When questioned concerning the safety of aspartame, the FDA

proclaims that it is "the most-studied product in history." Just how much trust should you place in this statement? What has been learned in these studies about the safety of aspartame? And what have been the actual experiences of the consumers who have used aspartame since its FDA approval and introduction as a sweetener?

ASPARTAME: HARMFUL DRUG OR SAFE SWEETENER?

In 1965 a chemist with the G.D. Searle Company was trying to develop a drug for ulcers. He was experimenting with two amino acids, phenylalanine and aspartic acid. These are only two of the numerous amino acids that the body normally uses in building proteins. Dr. Woodrow Monte, a nutrition scientist, writes that these two amino acids are

> found in natural proteins, and under normal circumstances are beneficial, if not essential for health. Proteins are complex molecules which contain many chemically bonded amino acids. It takes several enzymes to break these bonds and liberate the amino acids. This is a slow process and the amino acids are released gradually into the bloodstream. The quaternary structure of protein also slows the digestion of these amino acids; the amino acids in the center of the protein molecule aren't released until the outer layers of amino acids on the surface have been swept away. This natural time release process saves the body from large numbers of any one of these 21 amino acids being released into the bloodstream at any one time.[1]

Aspartic acid acts as an "excitatory" neurotransmitter in the brain. It functions as a chemical messenger, stimulating the neurons in the brain to "fire." Too much aspartic acid, as well as too much phenylalanine, entering the brain will cause the brain to get out of balance with the inhibitory amino acids, therefore interfering with normal brain function and possibly causing severe brain damage. Dr. Julian Whitaker suggests, "This is a likely reason why aspartame lowers the threshold of seizures, mood disorders, and other nervous system problems. This altered brain chemistry may also be responsible for the addictive nature of aspartame. Some patients report that getting off diet soda takes more willpower than giving up cigarettes!"[2]

Searle's research chemist next added methyl alcohol to his chemical mixture. This is the wood alcohol that was consumed by college students in the 1920s. In quantity, it can cause blindness, brain damage, and death. Inside the human body methyl alcohol breaks down into methanol, a nervous system toxin that can be extremely harmful to the optic nerve. Methanol is rapidly released into the bloodstream, where it is metabolized into other harmful metabolites, including formaldehyde and formic acid. Formaldehyde is embalming fluid and is a known carcinogen. Formic acid is the poison that ants inject into you when they bite. Its primary use in industry is for dyeing and finishing textiles.

The chemist then happened to lick his hand, and upon tasting the synthetic drug for ulcers, which was intended to be used in very small amounts and only when prescribed by a physician, he discovered that it was intensely sweet. Aspartame, the sweetener, was born!

Searle initially advertised that aspartame was "as natural as milk and bananas." Many of you may remember the ads well. The ads showed cows grazing in a green pasture and bunches of ripe yellow bananas. The ads also stated that the basic ingredients in aspartame were as natural as cow's milk and bananas.

Some doctors and scientists, who became familiar with the research, the initial consumer health complaints, and the perceived potential for harm, complained. They were quickly silenced. The FDA and the Federal Trade Commission allowed Searle to continue its advertising campaign. After a while, Searle quietly removed the ads. Aspartame and its derivatives would soon begin to appear everywhere and in everything.

WE HAVE BEEN BEGUILED AND DECEIVED

I believe there is a fascinating similarity between the introduction of aspartame into the American diet and the Biblical story of how Satan deceived Eve and persuaded her to partake of the fruit of the Tree of Knowledge of Good and Evil. Pause for a moment and read Chapters 1 and 2 in the Book of Genesis in the Bible. Whether or not you accept the Bible as true, the patterns of the two events are worth comparing. In Chapter 2, Verses 8 and 9, God explains to Moses that He placed the man Adam in a garden that He had planted eastward in Eden. The garden had contained a variety of trees, which both were pleasant to the sight and produced fruit that was good for food. In the midst or center of the garden He had also planted the Tree of Life and the Tree of Knowledge of Good and Evil.

In Verses 15 through 17, God explains how he had instructed Adam to take care of the garden. He had informed Adam that he could eat freely of the fruit of every tree in the garden except the Tree of Knowledge of Good and Evil. He told Adam that on the day he ate thereof, he would surely die. Adam's body had been formed in such a fashion that he was not subject to death. The chemicals contained within the forbidden fruit would change that condition, however. The molecular structure of his physical body would, over time, be altered and his cells would experience deterioration and death. Adam would become subject to death.

God then created Eve to be Adam's "help meet," and she became his wife (Verses 18 through 24). In Verses 1 through 6 of Chapter 3, the serpent, who is more crafty or sly than any other animal, approached Eve. Lucifer spoke to Eve through the mouth of the cunning serpent and asked, "Has God said that ye shall not eat of every tree of the garden?" Eve replied that they could eat of every tree except the Tree of Knowledge of Good and Evil, which was in the midst of the garden. She added that they were not even allowed to touch the fruit "lest ye die." The serpent responded, "Ye shall not surely die" but "your eyes shall be opened, and ye shall be as the gods knowing good and evil." Who could resist that?

While they conversed, Satan and his willing serpent accomplice must have lured Eve to the tree in the midst of the garden. In your mind's eye you can see the crafty serpent moving stealthily among the branches touching, caressing, and then eating the fruit. He did not immediately die. Now his words appeared to Eve to be very wise. "And when the woman saw that the tree was good for food, and that it was pleasant to the eyes, and a tree to be desired to make one wise, she took of the fruit thereof, and did eat, and gave also unto her husband with her; and he did eat." When the Lord approached them and asked if they had partaken of the fruit, Adam confessed that he had eaten of the fruit given him by Eve. Asked what she had done, Eve replied, "The serpent beguiled me, and I did eat."

To Eve the Lord said, "I will greatly multiply thy sorrow and thy conception; in sorrow thou shalt bring forth children. . . ." He told Adam that he would now have to work for their food until the day they died and their physical bodies returned to the dust of the earth (Verses 7 through 16). And so in innocently partaking of a fruit that was sweet to the taste, and which they had been told would make them wise, they caused the seeds of death to be sown within their bodies. Like the beguiling serpent, Adam and Eve did not die immediately. Although it took many years for the cells of their bodies to become fully corrupted, the forbidden fruit did eventually kill them. Eve was beguiled by the crafty advertising campaign instituted by Satan and carried out by the serpent.

When we compare the manner in which aspartame and its derivatives have been advertised, and what the results have been, with the way Satan introduced the forbidden fruit to our totally innocent, and unsuspecting, first parents, I believe the similarity is striking.

THE SEEDS OF ILLNESS AND DEATH

The current formulation of aspartame is 50 percent phenylalanine, 40 percent aspartic acid, and 10 percent methyl alcohol, creating a tiny molecule. One liter (about a quart) of most aspartame-containing drinks have 550 milligrams of aspartame. This yields 275 milligrams of phenylalanine, 220 milligrams of aspartic acid, and 55 milligrams of methanol. Some brands of diet soft drinks contain as much as four times more aspartame than other brands. According to the *Federal Register* of February 22, 1984, orange-flavored beverages tend to contain a much greater amount—up to 333 milligrams of aspartame per 12 fluid ounces. That adds up to 930 milligrams per liter!

Dr. Roberts, a true expert on the effects of aspartame on the human body, writes:

> Promotional material for aspartame implies that the body treats aspartame's two amino acids no differently than if they were derived from fruit, vegetable, milk or meat. During his testimony before the U.S. Senate hearing on aspartame on November 3, 1987, Dr. Frank Young, FDA Commissioner, emphasized that the amino acids in aspartame are metabolized in the same way as "natural" building blocks of protein. I disagree. There are profound differences in both the rates of digestion and the degree of absorption depending on whether these amino acids are provided by food or by aspartame. The usual forms of protein (such as meat) contain four or five percent phenylalanine . . . not 50 percent, as does aspartame. Moreover, [the phenylalanine contained in natural food sources is] slowly digested within the gastrointestinal tract, and in tandem with other neutral amino acids. This precludes an unbalanced flooding of the system with single amino acids. The situation is quite different with aspartame, where the body is suddenly deluged with large amounts of two amino acids.[3]

In addition, Dr. Roberts points out that consuming aspartame in a liquid form results in higher blood levels of the two amino acids than a powdered form would produce. However, most of the studies performed with aspartame have involved giving it in a capsule form. These studies, though controlled and double-blinded, were performed with a totally different product, different methodology, and different rate of assimilation than what is encountered by real people. Therefore, in my opinion, they provide little, if any, meaningful safety data.

Furthermore, these studies generally used nonheated aspartame-containing products such as a pudding that was freshly prepared just before being given to the test subjects. For example, in tests with thirty preschool boys that showed aspartame did not disrupt normal behavior, the aspartame was served in cold drinks, added as a syrup that had been kept refrigerated, and packed in crushed ice. In real life these boys would have ingested soft drinks that had been stored in warehouses and shipped in trucks for long periods of time and often at high temperatures.[4] According to the *Federal*

Register of July 8, 1983, aspartame shows a spoilage of 38 percent at 86°F and of over 50 percent at 104°F.

Correct information is the antecedent of knowledge, and the correct application of knowledge is the prerequisite of wisdom, the possession of which enables us to make intelligent choices. Therefore, it is important to understand the three components of aspartame and the effects that phenylalanine, aspartic acid, and methyl alcohol exert upon the structure and functions of the human body right down to the cellular level when they are consumed as aspartame.

Phenylalanine

As we discussed in Chapter 4, people with phenylketonuria, or PKU, lack the enzyme phenylalanine hydroxylase and therefore are unable to metabolize phenylalanine and convert it into other important amino acids. High concentrations of phenylalanine can pass through the so-called blood-brain barrier and cause severe brain damage. The concern is that PKU patients, and anyone else under certain conditions, can experience a significant elevation of phenylalanine in their blood resulting in damage to their brain cells. Dr. Roberts expresses deep concern regarding this possibility:

> The effects of entry of aspartame breakdown products into the brain may be even greater than currently believed. Studies on the neurotoxicity of aspartate and glutamate, a related compound, have demonstrated that several regions of the brain lack a so-called blood-brain barrier, which inhibits passage of certain substances into the brain. As a result, aspartame and other substances, including monosodium glutamate (MSG), can penetrate the brain freely, and selectively exert toxic effects.[5]

Russell L. Blaylock, M.D., professor of neurosurgery at the Medical University of Mississippi, agrees with Dr. Roberts. In his book *Excitotoxins: The Taste That Kills,* he explains that aspartate and glutamate are neurotransmitters normally found in the brain and spinal cord. However, he states that when aspartate reaches certain levels, attained when drinking a dozen diet sodas in a day or several packets of aspartame in a beverage, brain neurons are destroyed. Could this, as suggested by Dr. Blaylock and other physicians, be the cause of the seeming epidemic of the early onset of diseases such as Alzheimer's, Parkinson's, lupus, brain lesions and tumors, epilepsy, memory loss, and multiple sclerosis?

We must also note that high concentrations of phenylalanine are found in people with chronic kidney failure. Are high levels of phenylalanine a cause or an effect? Also, the absence of sufficient insulin in the blood may cause an increase in the level of phenylalanine. Insulin stimulates the synthesis of phenylalanine hydroxylase. This should be of profound concern to diabetics, who are led to believe that aspartame is not harmful to them. Further, by ingesting aspartame-containing soft drinks with foods rich in carbohydrates and poor in protein, such as desserts, many of which now also contain aspartame, one can significantly increase and even double the amount of phenylalanine in the brain. Research has documented that phenylalanine has the highest affinity for transport across the blood-brain barrier of all the circulating amino acids. When this increase occurs, the brain concentrations of the amino acid–derived neurotransmitters can be altered.[6] The question must then be posed: What is the level of destruction to the brain cells of children and teenagers who drink diet beverages containing aspartame while they eat pastries, candy, or other "sweets"?

Dr. Roberts reports:

> Flooding the brain with phenylalanine, the precursor of dopamine and norepinephrine, can radically affect brain neurotransmitters. The marked rise of brain phenylalanine following aspartame ingestion—with subsequent modification of norepinephrine, epinephrine and serotonin synthesis—also reflects a reduction of neutral amino acids (Wurtman 1985). An excess of certain neurotransmitters (for example, glutamate) is known to over stimulate certain populations of nerve cells in the brain . . . even causing their destruction.
>
> . . . Too much phenylalanine tends to "handicap the nutritional flow of amino acids to the brain" (Christensen 1987). Clinical expressions of this condition include a lowering of the seizure threshold in susceptible individuals, and altered mechanisms regulating hunger and satiety (Blundell 1986).[7]

That is, it is the underlying cause of significant fat gain and the occurrence of seizures.

This research has aptly demonstrated that too much of either aspartic acid or phenylalanine circulating in the blood can cause seizures and severe damage to the brain. What, then, is the potential harm to the brain when one significantly increases the blood level of both these amino acids by ingesting aspartame or its derivative products? Remember that aspartame is 50 percent phenylalanine, 40 percent aspartic acid, and 10 percent methyl alcohol.

Children and developing fetuses are at especially high risk. The potential for brain damage is at its greatest during these periods of maximum development and growth. Dr. Roberts reports that a scientist named Fisher demonstrated in 1971 that a fivefold increase in plasma phenylalanine concentration can impair brain function in the developing fetus and in children. This suggests that pregnant women who eat and drink products containing aspartame may produce children with mental impairment. Could this be a root cause of the apparent inability to concentrate and to learn, as well as the horrible and destructive abnormal behavioral traits, so rampant in much of today's youth? Could the multigenerational ingestion of these products, with the unavoidable deterioration of brain cells, be the underlying cause of the loss of normal, natural affection of one human being for another? Could the results of this brain damage be one of the underlying causes of a future world plague, as prophesied by John the Revelator in Revelation 16?

Could anything be more obvious? I believe no pregnant woman should ever eat or drink any product containing aspartame or its consumer derivatives.

Fisher also reported, "Brain function deterioration associated with increased concentrations of phenylalanine and other amino acids also occurs in patients with liver failure."[8]

It is important to be aware that aspartame and its various consumer products are not the only culprits that are potentially reeking havoc within the brains of consumers. Phenylalanine is appearing in numerous over-the-counter products widely advertised for the relief of arthritis, depression, migraine, dyslexia, obesity, alcoholism, and even whiplash. Dr. Roberts reports that people who experience adverse reactions to aspartame may have even worse reactions to these over-the-counter medications. In this day of worldwide distribution of medicines and processed foods that contain harmful ingredients, it has become mandatory that you read the labels of all products before consuming them or putting them upon your body.

Aspartic Acid

· The aspartame molecule is 40 percent aspartic acid. While aspartic acid is important in the metabolic process, it becomes harmful at excessive amounts. Eating carbohydrates or protein decreases the rise of aspartic acid in the blood. When aspartame-containing beverages that have no protein or carbohydrates are consumed, the potential result is a higher absorption and concentration of aspartic acid in the blood. "Under conditions of excess absorption it has caused endocrine disorders in mammals with markedly elevated plasma levels of luteinizing hormone and testosterone in the rat and release of pituitary gonadotropins and prolactin in the rhesus monkey," reports Dr. Monte. "The amount of luteinizing hormone in the blood is a major determinant of menstrual cycling in the human female."[9] Does this mean that aspartame may be the actual cause of the menstrual problems being experienced by American women in recent years?

Dr. Roberts reports that several studies offer evidence of the neurotoxicity of excess levels of aspartic acid, especially when consumed with foods to which glutamate and MSG have been added. "Some infants lack the enzyme required to metabolize aspartic acid," he says. "Moreover, the neurotoxic effects of aspartate and glutamate appear to be addictive." He lists five potential points that should be considered by consumers:

1. Aspartate and glutamate form up to 30 percent of the total free amino acid content of the brain.

2. Since severe confusion and memory loss are common reactions among individuals sensitive to aspartame, it is especially noteworthy that Alzheimer's patients show markedly diminished aspartate binding in their brain cells.

3. The chemical structure and transport system of aspartic acid are very similar to those of glutamic acid (glutamate), and research has already shown the toxicity of MSG.

4. D-aspartic acid has been shown to accumulate in the brain as it ages, possibly contributing to Alzheimer's disease and other brain disorders.

5. D-aspartate binding has been shown to be reduced in the brains of Alzheimer's patients.

Dr. Roberts suggests that the breakdown products of aspartame, other than its two amino acids and methanol, may also contribute to the numerous adverse reactions experienced by its users. "Dr. Jeffrey Bada, a University of California (San Diego) professor of chemistry and researcher at the Amino Acid Dating Laboratory of the Scripps Institution of Oceanography, has made significant contributions in this field," according to Dr. Roberts. "He detected up to ten different breakdown products of aspartame." These metabolites, he says, are released through "heating, prolonged storage, and interactions with other chemicals" in the food or beverage to which the sweetener has been added.[10]

The great alarm here is that people consume the greatest amounts of soft drinks containing aspartame during the hot summer months. This is the very time of greatest danger because the beverages are stored in hot warehouses for prolonged periods and are transported in unrefrigerated trucks. The internal temperatures within these metal trucks, with the summer sun beating down upon them, become extremely high. The temperatures within closed trucks and cars can easily exceed 150°F.

Conversely, in the wintertime people add aspartame directly to hot drinks, such as coffee and hot chocolate. Roberts reports that phenylalanine and aspartic acid in aspartame break down at room temperature when added to hot chocolate.

Methyl Alcohol

Methyl alcohol, also called wood alcohol, is a metabolic poison. It is the substance used to make antifreeze for car radiators. Because aspartame is 10 percent methyl alcohol, it is important to understand the effects of this highly toxic substance within the human body. Ingesting even moderate quantities of it can cause serious damage to living tissues, including blindness and even death. Among the patient-reported symptoms of methyl alcohol poisoning are lethargy, confusion, impaired articulation, leg cramps, back pain, severe headache, abdominal pain, labored breathing, vertigo, and visual loss. The symptoms reported by the Public Health Service include damage to the pancreas, liver, kidneys, heart, and lungs, as well as headache, ear buzzing, dizziness, nausea, difficulty walking, gastrointestinal disturbances, weakness, vertigo, chills, memory lapses, numbness, shooting pains in the extremities, behavioral disturbances, visual disturbances, and neuritis.[11]

Periodically the newspapers report an injury or death caused by drinking a substance containing methyl alcohol. Several years ago twenty-five persons in Italy died after drinking a table wine containing 5.7 percent methyl alcohol. In 2000, one teen was killed and eleven were injured when they drank a soda pop laced with methyl alcohol.

It is highly unusual to find methanol, the breakdown product of methyl alcohol, in nature. In its free form—that is, not locked or bound to another compound—methanol is usually produced or extracted from other substances. When ingested in foods or beverages, it is generally released within hours following consumption. Dr. Monte reports:

> Absorption in primates is hastened considerably if the methanol is ingested as free methanol as it occurs in soft drinks after the decomposition of aspartame during storage or in other foods after being heated. Regardless of whether the aspartame-derived methanol exists in food in its free form or still esterified to phenylalanine, 10 percent of the weight of aspartame intake of an individual will be absorbed by the bloodstream as methanol within hours after consumption.[12]

In addition, according to Dr. Monte, methyl alcohol syndrome occurs only in humans. Simply stated, humans do not possess the enzymes required to process methyl alcohol as do most of the animals commonly used in studies, such as monkeys, rats, rabbits, and dogs. The human digestive process is different from that of these animals. Dr. Mowrey was correct—humans are different from rats. Rats can ingest nine times more methyl alcohol than humans before showing symptoms. For these test animals, ethyl alcohol, which for humans is much less harmful than methyl alcohol, is more toxic than methyl alcohol. When one understands these facts, it is obvious that the testing of aspartame with rats yields little, if any, meaningful data concerning the safety of its ingestion by humans.

Further, the human body attempts to detoxify itself of methanol by oxidizing it to formaldehyde, then to formate or formic acid, and finally to carbon dioxide, which is exhaled. This requires a long period of time, however. It takes the body five times longer to eliminate methyl alcohol than it takes to rid itself of ethyl alcohol. As a matter of fact, ethanol is the classic antidote for methanol toxicity. Ethanol inhibits the metabolism of methanol and allows the body time for clearance of the toxin through the lungs and kidneys. In natural food sources, ethanol is found in concentrations of 5 to 500,000 times that of methanol.

Note that formaldehyde itself is a known carcinogen that is difficult to remove from the human body.[13] It often causes damage in the body even before its presence can be detected by medical laboratory analysis of body fluids or tissue.

We have reviewed only a very small portion of the vast amount of scientific information available concerning the harmful effects of aspartame upon the human body. Of the ninety-one studies performed by nonindustry-funded laboratories and available to the FDA in its decision-making process, eighty-four identified problems with consuming aspartame. In his *Health & Healing Newsletter,* Dr. Julian Whitaker reports:

> In the intervening years safety concerns have mushroomed. Ralph G. Walton, MD, Professor of Psychiatry at Northeastern Ohio

Universities College of Medicine, reviewed all the studies on aspartame and found 166 with relevance for human safety. Every one of the 74 studies funded by the aspartame industry gave it a clean bill of health, while 92 percent of those independently funded revealed safety problems.[14]

The doctor concludes this article by pleading with his readers to take his warning seriously:

> Although some people are much more sensitive to aspartame's adverse effects than others, damage is likely accumulative. Aspartame is particularly harmful to children and the developing fetus. I strongly urge anyone with an aspartame "habit" to get off this harmful sweetener.[15]

He suggests that people switch to stevia to "sweeten hot tea, coffee, yogurt, and other foods."[16]

Unfortunately, the ungreased wheels of change, carrying the weight of status quo, lumber incredibly slowly. That which is, often becomes the primary reason for keeping it that way. Change is never easy and often upsets the apple cart for numerous people and organizations. When change, even if for the best good of the people, causes a redirection of the flow of cash, monumental obstructions will appear to block or at least to impede the progress until the "right" individuals and organizations can take full advantage of the new course. We can only hope that in the end, truth will win out and justice prevail.

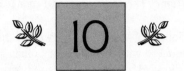

10

The FDA Stands Firmly Behind Aspartame

"Truth is a knowledge of things. In other words, it is an internal mental understanding or grasping of the way things really are; it is the subjective accurately reflecting the objective, the personal correctly reflecting the real, the map truly reflecting the territory."
—Stephen R. Covey, *The Divine Center* (Bookcraft, 1982)

As Jesus stood in the hall of judgment, Pontius Pilate, the Roman governor of Judea, asked Him, "What is truth?" Unfortunately, he didn't wait for an answer. Had he done so, perhaps much in this world might have been different. Jesus would have explained that truth never changes; it is always the same. As truth is today, so was it in the past, and so shall it be tomorrow, and a thousand years into the future. Only man spins "truth" to coincide with his own misunderstanding of evidence, and for his own selfish purposes.

In a court of law, witnesses swear an oath to tell the truth, the whole truth, and nothing but the truth. Lawyers present the truth as their clients see it and as they want it to be seen by others. I believe that lawyers and politicians value legal maneuvering above truth and justice.

Many scientists live in a paradigm in which they assert that truth is merely what they say it is. For them, today's definition is different from what it was yesterday and from what it will be tomorrow. They build today's "truth" based on the assumptions that they agreed upon yesterday. Many of them have not yet comprehended the reality that the laws of physics and nature do not change. What man understands to be a true law of nature or physics today may well be superceded by a higher law at some time in the future. The "law" or truth of things as they really are has not changed. Truth remains constant. It is only our perception, our comprehension of the laws of nature, and our ability to utilize the laws that have changed.

Truth cannot be clouded by half-truths, misrepresentations, or facts twisted to create new meanings. When I reached dating age, my mother told me that when I returned from a date or from being with friends, she would ask me what I had done. She told me that I must always tell the truth. Then she wisely added, "You don't have to tell me all of the truth but be sure that what you tell me is the truth." With this latitude, I cannot remember ever telling my parents a lie but I did not necessarily always tell them everything I knew.

For a youth, confronted with all of the trials and situations of adolescence, such freedom of expression and reporting of activity is perhaps necessary. However, in the world of science and medicine, it cannot be tolerated. The whole truth must prevail. We all have a right to know all of the facts, and the consequences thereof. In this book, I have tried to present the subjective objectively. My intent is to present you with both of the maps and allow you to choose your own route. The desired end of your journey is the happiness that comes from good health. Choose wisely.

THE FDA SPEAKS FOR ITSELF

In 1985, the FDA began a monitoring program to collect information about adverse reactions to food ingredients. In 1988, it published the results up to that date. According to the *FDA Consumer,* the FDA received 6,000 total complaints, of which 80 percent, or 4,800 complaints, were against aspartame. About 15 percent of the complaints were against sulfites, and 5 percent concerned MSG, food colorings, nitrites, other additives, and vitamin supplements.[1]

The FDA banned sulfite preservatives for use on fresh fruits and vegetables in August 1986. It banned many other products, especially in the "dietary supplement" category, after only a few complaints. What is the FDA's position regarding the complaints about aspartame? In so many words, it has been, and continues to be: "These people don't know what they are talking about. The FDA approved aspartame and it is safe for human consumption. The alleged complaints are without merit." It still proclaims aspartame to be "the most-studied product in history," and has designated it as GRAS, "generally regarded as safe."

Notwithstanding the FDA's adamant declarations of denial, the list of people who experience ill effects from this chemical product continues to grow. The original 4,800 people, and the thousands more (or doctors on their behalf) who have complained since 1988, report that they suffer from headache, anxiety, depression, and dizziness, including problems maintaining their balance. They suffer changes in mood and/or personality, extreme irritability, confusion, memory loss, severe slurring of the speech, and tremors comparable to those experienced by Parkinson's patients. They complain of nausea and vomiting, heart palpitations, cramps and severe abdominal pain, bloody stools, diarrhea, burning on urination, increased frequency of urination, excessive thirst, joint pain, fatigue and weakness, seizures and convulsions, slurred speech, decreased tear production, vision impairment, including pain in one or both eyes, and even total blindness. They complain of sleep difficulties, hyperactivity, shortness of breath, chest pains, ringing or buzzing in the ears, rashes, numbness or tingling in the extremities, hives, and loss of hair. Women complain of marked menstrual changes. In general, women appear to be more susceptible to the harmful effects of aspartame than men.

When the complainants stop using the product, the symptoms go away, returning only when they resume use of aspartame or products containing it. Many physicians refer to these symptoms as "aspartame disease." Some physicians and scientists believe it to be an underlying cause of brain tumors, comas, and death. The manufacturer of aspartame and the FDA deny any association between aspartame and these conditions. In fact, their oft-repeated response is that it is merely coincidental or a natural occurrence of spontaneous remission that the symptoms disappear when the patient stops ingesting aspartame-containing products.

In 1981 the FDA published this statement:

Three years after the cyclamate ban, G.D. Searle & Co., Skokie, Ill., petitioned the FDA [on March 5, 1973] to approve aspartame's use as a sweetener for table use: as a tablet for hot beverages, for use in cold cereals; as a dry base sweetener for powdered beverages, instant coffee and tea, gelatins, puddings, fillings, and dessert toppings; and as a flavoring agent in chewing gum.

Aspartame also has the same food value—four calories to the gram—as regular sugar, so its main appeal to calorie-conscious Americans lies in the fact that it is about 180 times sweeter than ordinary table sugar. A teaspoon of sugar has 18 calories; aspartame would provide only one-tenth of a calorie for the same amount of sweetness in a teaspoon of sugar. Saccharin, however, is 10 times sweeter than aspartame, but one of aspartame's appeals is that it has no bitter after-taste.

Also discovered accidentally—by a Searle scientist in 1965 who was doing research on new ulcer drugs—aspartame is a synthetic compound comprised of two amino acids, L-aspartic acid and the ethyl ester of L-phenylalanine. Unlike the other two sweeteners, aspartame was a new food additive that came under the full purview of the 1958 food additive legislation and, therefore, required pre-market clearance. FDA approved the Searle petition on July 26, 1974, for the uses described above, but challenges over the substance's safety and the validity of the company's data prevented the chemical from ever being marketed. At issue was whether aspartame, either alone or together with glutamate, posed a risk of contributing to mental retardation, brain damage, or to causing undesirable effects on the neuroendocrine systems, and whether the sweetener might cause brain neoplasms in rats.

There was agreement among all the parties involved to conduct a formal hearing before a scientific board of inquiry, which would then make a recommendation to the FDA Commissioner on whether to approve or disapprove aspartame. But before that board could convene, another problem arose. Questions were raised about the authenticity of certain animal studies conducted for Searle, and FDA wanted to resolve this issue before proceeding with the hearing. The company agreed to fund an independent review of the aspartame data by an outside group of pathologists.

On July 15, 1981, the new Commissioner of FDA, Dr. Arthur Hull Hayes Jr., announced the approval of aspartame. He based his approval on the board's findings, recommendations by FDA's Bureau of Foods, and the independent review of Searle's data. Dr. Hayes found the product to be safe at expected levels of consumption, as well as at the highest conceivable levels. (FDA will require the manufacturer to monitor consumption levels.)

The approval of aspartame opened a new chapter in the continuing saga of artificial sweeteners.[2]

A few pertinent facts were omitted from this FDA presentation. First, there is no mention that aspartame is 10 percent methanol. Thus, the fact is hidden that the product releases one molecule of methanol into the bloodstream for every molecule of aspartame consumed.[3] Second, there is no mention that the required formal hearing by the scientific board of inquiry ever took place. No report has ever been made available. Third, there is no mention that, not long after the FDA, under Dr. Hayes's commissionership, approved aspartame over the objections of FDA scientists, Dr. Hayes left the agency to become a $1,000-a-day consultant with Burston-Marsteller, the public relations firm for G.D. Searle.[4] (In 1981, this was a very high consulting fee—and it still is!) Dr. Hayes has never permitted himself to be interviewed concerning this matter. Fourth, there is no explanation offered for the statement that "Dr. Hayes found the product to be safe at expected levels of consumption. . . ." What are the "expected levels of consumption"? What are the "highest conceivable levels" of consumption? How could he have possibly known how much aspartame and its derivatives people would consume? Did he perform secret scientific tests himself that refuted the conclusions reached by the majority of the scientists? Finally, there is no explanation of how the FDA would require the manufacturer to monitor the consumption levels. Has the FDA followed through on this requirement? Where are the published reports?

What did Commissioner Hayes really mean by his statement regarding aspartame, made in the *Federal Register* in 1981, that "few compounds have withstood such detailed testing and repeated close scrutiny, and the process through which aspartame has gone should provide the public with additional confidence of its safety."[5]

The FDA statement indicates that Hayes relied upon the recommendation of the FDA's Bureau of Foods. Subsequently, in 1985, Dr. Stanford Miller, chief of the FDA's Bureau of Foods, explained to a U.S. Senate hearing: "I don't know of any substance in recent years that has been looked at with the scrutiny of aspartame. No one has yet come up with the slightest evidence to show that we were wrong in approving it."[6] Consequently, aspartame became touted by the manufacturer, the FDA, and other supporters as "the most thoroughly tested additive in history." Tested it was, but is it really safe? Read Dr. Miller's last sentence again.

Two years later, on November 3, 1987, FDA Commissioner Dr. Frank Young reported to a Senate hearing: "In conclusion, we do not have any medical or scientific evidence that undermines our confidence in the safety of aspartame. This confidence is based on years of study, analysis of adverse reactions, and research in the scientific community, including studies supported by the FDA."[7]

Is it possible that these FDA officials had consumed so much aspartame that they had contracted "aspartame disease" and that it rendered them both blind and deaf or caused them to lose all sense of reason due to brain cell alteration? Were they aware only of the studies performed by G.D. Searle? Did they not read the eighty-four negative studies performed by independent nonindustry-funded laboratories?

All humor aside, of primary interest to every American is the answer to this question: How can the FDA safeguard the health and safety of American citizens while being influenced by the very corporations it is supposed to regulate? Following a lengthy investigation, freelance writer Bill Strubbe wrote an eye-opening account of what went on among the FDA, other government agencies, and the manufacturer of aspartame. According to his findings, within several years of aspartame being approved and flooding the consumer market, a number of FDA and government officials left their positions "and took jobs closely linked to the food, beverage, and NutraSweet industries."[8]

Senator Howard Metzenbaum, who held Senate hearings on the dangers of aspartame in 1985, released documents disclosing that in the late 1970s, "two senior Justice Department prosecutors investigating criminal allegations against G.D. Searle & Co. for falsifying NutraSweet safety tests results, later joined the law firm of Sidney & Austin, which represented G.D. Searle during the lengthy criminal investigation." While I choose not to reveal the names of these government prosecutors, one of them, aware of the statute of limitations, delayed pursuing prosecution, thus placing Searle beyond the time limit for legal action.[9]

According to Strubbe, former Assistant U.S. Attorney Ed Johnson, who served under William Sessions (later director of the FBI) said, "The aspartame manufacturer has a lot of political influence, and when the FDA Director refused to allow aspartame on the market, he was replaced by one who would."[10]

Former FDA investigator Arthur Evangelista explained, "Though it's against ethics laws for an FDA official to sit in on any action regarding a firm with which they had any prior relationship there is nothing to stop federal officials from being influenced with promises of a position in a firm they are meant to be regulating." Strubbe reports that Evangelista suggested influence pedaling is a common practice at the FDA, as is the use of monies from political action committees to influence politicians, who in gratitude then use their influence on the regulatory agencies. Evangelista related a very telling account of two Texas agricultural inspectors whom he had recommended be charged for criminal cover-up and abuse of powers. "My FDA supervisor requested the charges be 'toned down' and then sat on the report. Later, I found him at the computer not only re-writing the endorsement of prosecution, but also part of my investigative notes and the report itself!" The FDA supervisor then placed the "final version" on Evangelista's desk for his signature with an accompanying note requesting that he "destroy all previous copies."[11]

"As the revolving door continues to spin," suggests Strubbe, "the potential for conflict of interest within the government agency comes into question. In 1999," when Monsanto was the parent company of NutraSweet, "Dr. Virginia Weldon, Vice President for Public Policy at Monsanto, was considered for the FDA's commissioner post. On June 14, 1999 retiring FDA Commissioner Michael

Friedman became the Senior Vice President for Clinical Affairs at G.D. Searle & Co.'s drug unit."[12]

Because the controversy about aspartame continued to rage, the FDA published the following statement in 1994:

> After reviewing scientific studies, FDA determined in 1981 that aspartame was safe for use in foods. In 1987, the General Accounting Office investigated the process surrounding FDA's approval of aspartame and confirmed the agency had acted properly. However, FDA has continued to review complaints alleging adverse reactions to products containing aspartame. To date, FDA has not determined any consistent pattern of symptoms that can be attributed to the use of aspartame, nor is the agency aware of any recent studies that clearly show safety problems.[13]

It is fascinating that the FDA called aspartame "the most-studied product in history" and completely safe for unlimited consumption, with 84 of 166 studies identifying safety concerns. At the same time it released the statement, it said that the more than 500 studies regarding stevia, of which only 4 were negative (and we discussed the total absurdity of them in Chapter 7), were insufficient to determine its safety. Had the death of brain neurons been that extensive?

In an "FDA Talk Paper" published in 1996, prepared by the Press Office to guide FDA personnel in responding to questions regarding aspartame, the agency stated, "The FDA stands behind its original approval decision, but the agency remains ready to act if credible scientific evidence is presented to it—as would be the case for any product approved by the FDA." It added, "In 1981 after extensive review of the record by FDA scientists, then Commissioner Arthur Hull Hayes approved aspartame as a food additive. In his decision Hayes noted that additional scientific data from a Japanese study about the brain tumor issue corroborated his decision. The [Public Board of Inquiry] chairman later wrote in a letter to Hayes that the data would have caused that panel to give aspartame an 'unqualified approval.'"

This statement raises three questions:

1. If one Japanese study was sufficient to motivate the FDA to give aspartame "unqualified approval" despite eighty-four negative studies, why, with dozens and dozens of Japanese studies proving the safety of stevia, does the FDA withhold approval of that substance?

2. Why does stevia enjoy a 52 percent market share in Japan as that country's primary commercial sweetener?

3. Why do the Japanese health authorities consider aspartame to be harmful?

The November-December 1999 issue of the *FDA Consumer* carried an article titled "Sugar Substitutes: Americans Opt for Sweetness and Lite." The sections of the article in which aspartame is discussed are extremely interesting. As you read the article, you might consider the question, is the author doing "damage control" for the FDA or is he secretly trying to warn readers, who can read between the lines, of the dangers of consuming aspartame?

Aspartame has come under fire in recent years from individuals who have used the Internet in an attempt to link the sweetener to brain tumors and other serious disorders. But FDA stands behind its original approval of aspartame, and subsequent evaluations have shown that the product is safe. A tiny segment of the population is sensitive to one of the sweetener's byproducts and should restrict intake. However, the agency continually monitors safety information on food ingredients such as aspartame and may take action to protect public health if it receives credible scientific evidence indicating a safety problem. . . .

While questions about saccharin may persist, the safety of another artificial sweetener, aspartame, is clearcut, say FDA officials. FDA calls aspartame, sold under trade names such as NutraSweet and Equal, one of the most thoroughly tested and studied food additives the agency has ever approved. The agency says the more than 100 toxicological and clinical studies it has reviewed confirm that aspartame is safe for the general population.

This message would not necessarily be apparent to consumers surfing the Internet, especially those who use Web-based search engines to find information about sugar substitutes or artificial sweeteners. Websites with screaming headlines and well-written text attempt to link aspartame consumption to systemic lupus, multiple sclerosis, vision problems, headache, fatigue, and even Alzheimer's disease. One report distributed nationally over e-mail systems claims that aspartame-sweetened soft drinks delivered to military personnel during the Persian Gulf War may have prompted Gulf War syndrome.

No way, says FDA, along with many other health organizations such as the American Medical Association. David Hattan, Ph.D., acting director of FDA's division of health effects evaluation, says there is "no credible evidence" to support, for example, a link between aspartame and multiple sclerosis or systemic lupus. Some Internet reports claim that patients suffering from both conditions went into remission after discontinuing aspartame use. "Both of these disorders are subject to spontaneous remissions and exacerbation," says Hattan. "So it is entirely possible that when patients stopped using aspartame they might also coincidentally have remission of their symptoms."

It is true, says Hattan, that aspartame ingestion results in the production of methanol, formaldehyde and formate—substances that could be considered toxic at high doses. But the levels formed are modest, and substances such as methanol are found in higher amounts in common food products such as citrus juices and tomatoes.

Other circulating reports claim that two amino acids in aspartame—phenylalanine and aspartic acid—can cause neurotoxic effects such as brain damage. "This is true in certain individuals and in high enough doses," says Hattan. He explains that a very small group of people who have the rare hereditary disease phenylketonuria, estimated at 1 in 16,000 people, are sensitive to phenylalanine. These "phenylalketonurics" have to watch their intake of phenylalanine from other sources as well. People with advanced liver disease and pregnant women with high levels of phenylalanine in the blood may also have trouble metabolizing the substance. FDA requires all products containing aspartame to be labeled for phenylalanine so consumers will be aware of the substance's presence and can avoid or restrict it.

Aspartic acid also has the potential to cause brain damage at very high doses. But under normal intake levels, the brain's mechanism for controlling aspartic acid levels ensures no adverse effects. It is unlikely that any consumer would eat or drink enough aspartame to cause brain damage: FDA figures show that most aspartame users only consume about 4 to 7 percent of the acceptable daily intake the agency has set for the sweetener.

Still other reports attempt to link aspartame to seizures and birth defects. Regarding seizures, Hattan cites animal and human studies showing that the sweetener neither causes nor enhances the susceptibility of seizures. Aspartame also has been evaluated for its potential to cause reproductive effects or birth defects. Again, researchers found no evidence, even in test animals fed the sweetener at doses much higher than those to which humans would be exposed.

Approved in 1981, aspartame is 180 times sweeter than sugar. It is used in products such as beverages, breakfast cereals, desserts, and chewing gum, and also as a tabletop sweetener. In 1996, a study raised the issue that aspartame consumption may be related to an increase in brain tumors following FDA's approval of the sweetener in 1981. But analysis of the National Cancer Institute's database on cancer incidence showed that cases of brain cancers began increasing in 1973—well before aspartame was approved— and continued to increase through 1985. In recent years, brain tumor frequency has actually decreased slightly. NCI currently is studying aspartame and other dietary factors as part of a larger study of adult brain cancer.[14]

This article also raises many concerns and questions. Consider a few of them. First, it implies that you should not believe information placed in the Internet—that you should place your total trust in the FDA, and believe only what that agency determines is correct. It is true that people put incorrect information on the Internet to deceive the unwary, but it contains more data that is truth. We must each discern truth from error. You must determine who put the information there and what their motivation is. Further, the article never mentions the numerous statements of harm made by medical doctors and scientists.

Second, the article states that 100 toxicological studies confirm the safety of aspartame. Why does the FDA not inform the public that 74 of these studies were performed by the manufacturer of aspartame or others in the industry who had a vested interest in the outcome of the research? Why does the FDA not inform the public that 84 out of 91 studies not funded by the aspartame industry found that there were indeed safety problems with the product and warned against its approval by the agency and consumption by humans? Why does it not mention that of the seven remaining studies (out of the 91), six were performed by the FDA, which might place them in the category of industry-sponsored studies?[15] Did the FDA review only the positive industry-funded studies?

Third, why does the FDA discount all of the harm experienced by thousands upon thousands of people and belittle their suffering? Why does the FDA reject the findings of the physicians who care for these people, record their symptoms, and monitor their response to the elimination of aspartame from their diet? If there is the slightest possibility that the dozens and dozens of illnesses and conditions enumerated above might be caused or exacerbated by aspartame, why is this not fully investigated by the FDA? Is this not the very reason for the existence of the FDA?

Fourth, could there be validity to the theory that aspartame-laden soft drinks were a cause of or at least a contributory factor to Gulf War syndrome? Why is this adamantly denied without any investigation? Remember what occurs to aspartame when it is stored in hot temperatures. The desert of Saudi Arabia is very hot and military personnel drank large amounts of aspartame in soft drinks that also contained no calories, thus, increasing the danger. Who is afraid of discovering the truth—whatever it may be?

Fifth, the FDA says "no way" to the Gulf War syndrome link to aspartame. Where is the research to substantiate this emphatic denial? Are we to believe it simply because the agency says it? Is this not the same agency that approved the drug thalidomide as safe for human use? This is the drug that caused such horrible birth defects. Babies were born without hands, feet, arms, or legs. But the FDA had proclaimed thalidamide to be safe. Who are we to believe?

Sixth, where is the research that proves "there is no credible evidence" to document an aspartame link to patients misdiagnosed with and treated for multiple sclerosis or systemic lupus, as proclaimed by David Hattan? Physicians who care for these patients say that at least some of them are misdiagnosed and are actually suffering from "aspartame disease." The cure is merely to stop consuming all the products that contain aspartame or any of its derivatives. The doctors and scientists do not say that aspartame *causes* multiple sclerosis or lupus; I believe Hattan misinterprets their findings. They state that for some people aspartame mimics the symptoms of these diseases. In my opinion, Hattan's statement that "it is entirely possible that when patients stopped using aspartame they might also have had remission of their symptoms" is foolish and unscientific.

Seventh, Hattan admits "that aspartame ingestion results in the production of methanol, formaldehyde and formate—substances that could be considered toxic at high doses. But the levels formed are modest, and substances such as methanol are found in higher amounts in common food products such as citrus juices and tomatoes." I believe these statements are true, but deceptive. (Remember the serpent's beguiling statement to Eve.) Are they based on ignorance or deceit? According to Dr. Woodrow Monte, a food scientist, methanol is a toxicant with no therapeutic properties. Just two teaspoons are considered a lethal dose for humans.[16] Dr. Monte also taught us that methanol studies using animals are without validity for human evaluation since the animals generally used for tests possess the biochemical pathways to detoxify themselves, while humans do not. We also learned that "ethanol, the classic antidote for methanol toxicity, is found in natural food sources of methanol at concentrations of 5 to 500,000 times that of the toxin. Ethanol inhibits metabolism of methanol and allows the body time for clearance of the toxin through the lungs and kidneys."[17] Natural food sources provide the antidote to methanol at the same time that it is ingested and, thus, protect man from its harmful effects. Aspartame does not offer this "saving grace."

It must also be noted that the reference used by the FDA concerning the presence of methanol in fruit and citrus juice is more than forty years old. Dr. Roberts writes that Hattan admitted to him in 1987 that he was not aware or any more recent analyses[18]—nor does he reference any in this article. However, it is now known that orange juice and grapefruit juice average as much as ten times more ethanol than methanol.[19] I believe these findings nullify Hattan's claim that the methanol in aspartame is no different from the methanol in citrus and tomatoes.

Eighth, Hattan, currently the acting director of the FDA's Division of Health Effects Evaluation, admits that phenylalanine and aspartic acid "in certain individuals and in high enough doses" can "cause neurotixic effects and brain damage." But, he says, "It is unlikely that any consumer would eat or drink enough aspartame to cause brain damage. FDA figures show that most aspartame users only consume about 4 to 7 percent of the acceptable daily intake the agency has set for the sweetener." How does he or the FDA know how much aspartame is consumed in a day, a week, or a month? Have they interviewed all 150 million users? Do they watch as children, teenagers, and adults guzzle down diet soft drinks and ingest the more than 9,000 products that contain aspartame? Has the FDA ever informed the general public about how much aspartame they can safely ingest? Is Hattan just blowing smoke to take the pressure off the FDA and aspartame?

Ninth, where is the FDA-required labeling on all products containing aspartame as a warning to people with phenylalanine problems?

And tenth, how can Hattan be so sure that aspartame is safe? It was this same David Hattan who, as chief of the Regulatory Affairs Staff at the FDA Office of Nutrition and Food Science, reluctantly provided Dr. Roberts with "a summary of the information up to July 1987 on 149 consumers with alleged aspartame-induced convulsions. It is noteworthy that the majority (87 percent) of reactions were classed as Type 1 (most severe category). The majority of these complainants also cited other aspartame-associated problems."[20] In my opinion, Dr. Hattan has known the dangers of aspartame use from the beginning and yet has stated, "The large body of animal and clinical research carried out in a controlled environment convinces me that aspartame is safe." Has everyone at the FDA played the ostrich and stuck his head into the sand—or the aspartame muck, as the case may be?

Fortunately there are a few courageous scientists who have spoken in opposition to the official FDA position. Dr. Jacqueline Verrett, a former FDA toxicologist and a member of the FDA task force, testified during a congressional investigation in 1985 that the safety tests were a "disaster" and should have been "thrown out." She said that the studies left many unanswered questions about possible birth defects and aspartame's safety. Regarding the aspartame safety tests conducted by Searle, Dr. Marvin Legator, professor of environmental toxicology at the University of Texas, said, "I've never seen anything as bad as Searle's" research. He labeled Searle's studies as "scientifically irresponsible and disgraceful."[21]

Dr. Richard Wurtman, a researcher at the Massachusetts Institute of Technology, reported in 1986 that he had been contacted by more than 100 persons who claimed to have experienced aspartame-associated seizures. He said that he was struck by the frequency of previous migraine headaches in these individuals. They noted that their headaches intensify prior to their convulsions. In 1987, Dr. Wurtman reported that his experiments indicated that aspartame in low doses enhances seizures in animals that are predisposed to unusual brain activity.[22]

At the Senate hearing held on August 1, 1985, Dr. M. Adrian Gross, then a senior FDA pathologist, asked, "In view of all these indications that the cancer-causing potential of aspartame is a matter that has been established way beyond any reasonable doubt, one can ask: 'What is the reason for the apparent refusal by the FDA to invoke for this food additive the Delaney Amendment to the Food, Drug, and Cosmetic Act?'"

In as early as 1981, Dr. Douglas L. Park, staff science advisor for the Office of Health Affairs, Department of Health and Human Services, concluded his assigned analysis of the Public Board of Inquiry (PBOI) hearings on the safety of aspartame relative to brain gliomas in rats. He stated, "I believe that aspartame has not been shown to be safe for the proposed food additive uses. Along with the Board of Inquiry, I must recommend, therefore, that aspartame not be approved until additional studies are carried out using proper experimental designs."

During the Senate hearing of August 1, 1985, Dr. Gross, in an attempt to prevent the licensing of aspartame, testified:

> I would view the Acceptable Daily Intake (ADI) set by the FDA for aspartame (50 mg/kg body weight/day) as totally unwarranted

and extremely high in that it can be associated with completely unacceptable risks as far as the induction of such (brain) tumors is concerned. It is clear that risks of this magnitude for what the FDA regards as a "safe" level of exposure to aspartame represents an outright calamity or disaster.[23]

In this same regard, Dr. W. M. Pardridge, author of scientific studies on the dangers of aspartame, stated in 1987 that the intake of 10 milligrams of aspartame per 1 kilogram of body weight regarded by aspartame researchers H. L. Levy and S. E. Waisbren (1987) as "large amounts" could be ingested by a 50-pound child as a single 12-ounce can of a carbonated diet drink.[24]

Dr. Verrett, again testifying before the Senate hearing on November 3, 1987, stated that she had found serious departures from standard procedures during her analysis of the original studies performed by Searle in the early 1970s. Uterine polyps, altered blood cholesterol, and other changes were discarded as "minor" findings. She said:

> It is unthinkable that any reputable toxicologist giving a complete objective evaluation of this data resulting from such a study could conclude anything other than that the study was uninterpretable and worthless and should be repeated. This is especially important for an additive such as aspartame, which, as we have heard already today is intended for and is now being used in such widespread and uncontrolled fashion.[25]

With regard to Searle's testing of the safety of aspartame, Dr. Alexander Schmidt, FDA commissioner from 1972 to 1976, was quoted as stating that it was "incredibly sloppy science."[26]

In the Senate hearing of August 1, 1985, Senator Metzenbaum stated, "The [Public Board of Inquiry] has not been presented with proof of a reasonable certainty that aspartame is safe for use as a food additive under its intended conditions for use."[27]

Dr. Roberts writes that the Government Accounting Office, reporting on its two-year investigation of aspartame, stated in July 1987 that more than half of the scientists it surveyed were concerned about the neurological reactions and other potential adverse effects of aspartame products in children. A total of 40 percent of these scientists called for further research, 32 percent sought new warnings, and 15 percent suggested a total ban.[28]

In light of all this, the FDA cannot find any scientific evidence that warrants further research on aspartame, or any reason to warn the public concerning possible danger from making this drug a part of their daily diet.

Where is the truth? Whom can you believe? As stated early on in this book, you are the judge and jury. The very lives of your loved ones, as well as your own, may depend upon your decision.

UNANSWERED HEALTH QUESTIONS CONCERNING ASPARTAME

Is it possible that aspartame-laden foods and beverages are the underlying or contributory cause of any of the following conditions?

- The attention deficit disorder problems exhibited in children, who now require harmful and expensive drugs to give temporary self-control

- The behavioral problems exhibited by grade school children, high school students, and adults, including professional athletes

- The apparent inability of many American high school students to learn

- The intellectual deterioration among Americans

- The diseases and conditions caused by the deterioration or death of brain cells

- The medical "mistakes" made by doctors and nurses in hospitals

- The pilot error–caused crashes of commercial and private aircraft

- The automobile accidents caused by inattention or vision problems

- The errors made by people in business and banking

- The inability to concentrate and complete projects

- Marital difficulties and divorce

- Frequent headaches

- Uncontrollable weight gain

In my opinion, the answer is yes.

The thought that aspartame could be a contributing factor in these and many additional conditions and events, and the numerous "diseases" possibly linked to it, may initially seem unreasonable. But is it? Review in your mind the things that reputable doctors, scientists, and consumers have discovered about this "most-studied product in history," so adamantly supported by the FDA. Is consuming this synthetic product really worth the risk? Remember, aspartame was developed by the G.D. Searle Company to be used for ulcers, to be dispensed by a pharmacist, authorized by the prescription of a medical doctor. It was to be used only for short periods of time. I believe aspartame is a drug being allowed to masquerade as a sweetener. Many physicians and scientists who have studied it state that it is a drug with severe side effects.[29,30]

These scientists and medical doctors have suggested the following: If you, or a family member, suffer from any of the symptoms, situations, or conditions enumerated for aspartame or its derivatives, stop all use of every product containing this chemical sweetener for a period of at least ninety days. This may not be an easy task. You will have to read the labels of all processed food and beverage products—*before* you buy them. The possible results are well worth the effort. If you experience improvement, you will have discovered the true cause of your suffering and anguish. The simplest solution may well be the easiest, and the least expensive. Try the experiment. It may change your life. It may greatly improve your health and increase your happiness and joy for living.

You may discover that for you, anything is better than aspartame—even stevia. Give stevia a try. You will be amazed at what this natural sweetener and healing herb can do for you, and for those you love.

Many people pray for healing, for improved health, and for well-being. But if they refuse to stop eating, drinking, applying, or smoking the very poison that causes their illness or impaired condition, on what basis can they expect God to cure them, or bless them with improved health and vitality?

The decision is yours. Do you want to continue using an "artificial sweetener" that is harmful to your body and brain, or do you prefer to use a natural product that is truly a miracle herb? Stevia, as we have learned, is not only intensely sweet, but also incredibly healing to the human body. Reread Chapters 1 through 3 concerning the numerous health-promoting benefits of this truly amazing herb that is both sweet to the taste and healing to the body. Then select the forms of stevia most suitable for the needs and desires of your family—and observe the improvement in the health and well-being of your loved ones.

Knowledge, enhanced with experience, reflection, and evaluation, will bring wisdom into your life.

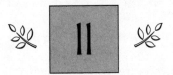

An Appointment with Destiny

"You can fool all of the people some of the time, and you can fool some of the people all of the time, but you can't fool all of the people all of the time."

—Abraham Lincoln

During the 1970s, my wife and I were forced to learn about the dangers aspartame posed for children with phenylketonuria in order to protect two of our children, Michael and Erin, from brain damage. I had no idea that the next decade would thrust me into a battle with the powerful companies that manufacture and market this artificial substance. I would come to view this industry as a fire-belching beast, eager to roast and devour anything and everyone who encroaches into what it considers to be its own private territory.

The artificial sweetener industry was not the only danger into which my innocent venture took me. Financially, the end of the 1970s and the first two years of the 1980s were good to me. A physician friend and I had opened dialysis centers on the Navajo reservation to fill a critical need of the Navajo in Arizona and New Mexico. We sold these centers to the same major hospital chain that purchased the dialysis services corporation of which I was president. My adventure into stevia's field of dreams would cause the loss of everything I owned except my home and automobile. However, even this was not the worst danger that lay ahead. Unknowingly, I was standing on the very edge of a precipice, and the slightest misstep could cause me to plunge over the edge to be lost for decades in the frightful dungeons of Paraguay.

IN TIMES OF PERIL

Beginning with my first trip to Paraguay in 1983, I met with government authorities and farmers in an effort to persuade them to increase the agricultural production of stevia and to establish processing facilities to extract the sweet glycosides from the leaves. I failed. Paraguay was poor, and neither the wealthy among its citizens nor its government officials were willing to take the financial risk. Besides, unknown to me at the time, H. H., the peace corps worker who had originally gotten me involved, had told government officials and the press that James A. May, a wealthy North American, was going to invest $10 million in American money to develop the stevia industry in Paraguay.

The announcement had been a feature story in the major newspaper in Asunción—before my arrival. It was a lie on all counts and H. H. knew it. He counted on the fact that my Spanish was poor, that I would never see the newspaper, and that I, therefore, would never know what he had done. Had I possessed $10 million to invest in stevia, it would have been a true statement. But I had no money. For him, however, as my self-publicized "official agent in Paraguay," this helped doors to open wide. He took every advantage to establish himself as someone of great importance to the economy of Paraguay.

A few years later, when I gained possession of his newspaper scrapbook and read the article, I understood why everyone, including farmers, businessmen, and even the president of Paraguay and his ministers of agriculture and commerce, were eager to meet with me. I had always wondered why these important officials had been so friendly and so very willing to be of service to me, just a poor, North American nobody. I was most surprised during my visit in May 1983 when I was informed that "His Supreme Excellency General Alfredo Stroessner," president of Paraguay, wanted to meet with me.

Presidente Stroessner's Bavarian father had settled in Paraguay in the 1890s. He had married a local girl and had established a brewery in a remote country town. In time the son had become a war hero—no small thing in a nation whose history had been written in fire and blood. Paraguay had gained its independence from Spain in 1811, after which it had fought terrible wars against the combined forces of Brazil, Argentina, and Uruguay. Between 1865 and 1870 nearly half the population had been killed. Only 28,000 adult men had survived the wars. Although a strongly Catholic nation, the local church hierarchy had tolerated the government policy of each man taking several "wives" and rebuilding the population. The church did not officially permit multiple marriages but it understood that polygamy was essential to the survival of the nation, and that human babies were the country's most important crop. To this day, the practice of polygamy lingers in some areas under only a very thin veil of secrecy.

Stroessner's time came in the 1930s, when Paraguay repeatedly clashed with Bolivia over a desolate wilderness, northwest of Asunción, called the Chaco. Another 100,000 men died winning this barren wilderness. Over the ensuing years, by intrigue and stealth, Stroessner rose to general and then seized power in a bloody coup in 1954. Three months later, he ran, without opposition, for president. The next three decades established that the only uncertainty in his election victories was the size of the majority of votes he would decide to allocate to himself.

In 1980, while the Nicaraguan dictator, Anastasio Somosa, was visiting Presidente Stroessner, he was assassinated by a Nicaraguan hit team in the center of Asunción, Paraguay's capitol city. He and his car were blown to bits by a rocket. The president immediately imposed a state of siege. Marshal law continued for years, with all civilian liberties suspended.

During my first few trips to Paraguay, I felt very intimidated when walking through the streets. Soldiers, armed with automatic weapons, were stationed every few yards. Since I was a "foreigner," my every move was watched closely. I was stopped repeatedly by the military police and required to produce my official documents, proving that I was in the country legally. I had been informed that their instructions, regarding anyone who appeared suspicious, were to shoot first and ask questions later. In time I became adjusted to the situation but I always remained cautious.

The morning of my scheduled meeting with the president, I received a phone call from his aide, who explained that due to a government emergency, "El Presidente" must postpone our meeting. He wanted to reschedule it for three days later. He could not comprehend my answer when I explained that I could not delay my return to America. How could I not be willing to delay my return in order to meet with the most powerful man in all of South America? He was totally stunned when my translator repeated in Spanish, "I promised my three sons that I would be home in time to take them on a church-sponsored father-and-son overnight outing." Having missed the previous year's outing as well as other activities with them because of work, I had given them my word that I would not miss this one. I could not break my promise to my little boys. There are priorities in life.

Perhaps keeping my word to my sons and not meeting Presidente Stroessner was truly a blessing. The following October, the *London Times,* in its Sunday supplement magazine, reported in a lengthy article about Stroessner that according to Amnesty International, there were usually between a few hundred and several thousand political prisoners locked away in Paraguay's jails at any one time. The article also said that there were numerous well-documented cases of prisoners being murdered in custody, with a number held, some in atrocious conditions, for up to twenty-five years without trial.

I have not permitted myself to contemplate what my fate might have been had I not kept my word of honor to my boys and had met with this powerful and vindictive ruler. What if he had learned that I did not have millions of American dollars to invest in the failing economy of Paraguay and that my self-proclaimed "official representative" in Paraguay had lied to the press, to members of his cabinet, and thus to him? It is not improbable that I would have found myself in one of Paraguay's feared prisons, where according to the *London Times* men were employed to torture and often kill the inmates. During one of my ensuing trips to Paraguay, I would be arrested for taking a photograph of the street intersection where I caught a city bus daily for the ride to the downtown printing company I had contracted to print product boxes and advertising. Working with a Guarani Indian artist in an office at the printing plant, I was designing the packaging and writing promotional materials. Only my friendship and association with the highly respected Colonel Luís Ramirez kept me out of prison. But that is another story for another time.

As I read the old newspaper articles, it became frightfully obvious that H. H. had translated neither my statements nor my questions accurately when I had met with the two enthusiastic ministers of government, the press, farmers, and businessmen. They all had thought that I was going to invest $10 million in Paraguay. The name I had chosen for the company had played right into his plans. I thought a corporate name such as United American Industries, Inc., with a product brand name of Wisdom of the Ancients, would exemplify cooperation and unity of purpose between our countries. The Paraguayans had interpreted it as a huge, wealthy North American corporation. Stevia was finally going to make them rich, they thought. Perhaps, over time, that could have been a possibility. However, the combined deceitfulness of many individuals and organizations turned their dream—and mine—into a nightmare.

For two years I sent every dollar I could scrape together to H. H. in order to buy the various herbs for the products we were going to produce and market in the United States. He owned and operated a Paraguayan company that was to purchase, process, and export the herbs to me. No matter how much money I sent to him, it was never enough. He always required more. He claimed that everything cost much more than we had originally projected. Later, I would learn that he had not spent all the money on buying the herbs, paying the artist, printing the packaging, and establishing his business structure. Most of it he had put toward maintaining the lifestyle that would portray his importance among the locals. When he finally fled Paraguay, he would tell others that he was leaving with a "ton of money." Apparently, I was not the only one he had duped.

I had found an investor in Arizona (both a friend and a surgeon) to help with the project but the money was draining fast. Before long H. H. would blindfold me and lead me to the edge of the quicksand. I suppose he believed that once I was buried beneath the surface, he would be left with the spoils. But that's a story for another time and place. For now, H. H. had me and the Paraguayans fooled, but it would not last for all time. I can be fooled only some of the time, not all of the time. Soon I would begin to see through the façade and into his deception.

Swords in Hand, Warriors Step Forth

The year 1994 was the turning point for stevia in its battle with the FDA and the fire-breathing beast that had so effectively kept it from American consumers. Journalists began to write about the sweet wonders of stevia. More physicians began to learn about the herb and to recommend it to their patients. U.S. congressmen, led by Senator Orrin Hatch of Utah, Senator Tom Harkin of Iowa, and Representative Bill Richardson of New Mexico, decided that the FDA had exceeded its boundaries.

These three members of Congress drew the weapon that would slightly wound the fierce dragon. Their sword was the word of law. After fierce political infighting, Congress passed the Dietary Supplement Health and Education Act (DSHEA), which was signed into law by President Clinton on October 25, 1994. Under the provisions of this law, herbal products could be marketed as dietary or nutritional supplements without first obtaining FDA approval as long as their manufacturers did not make any disease-fighting claims. Structure-function claims, however, were required to appear on the product labels. Sweet revenge!

Unfortunately, our opportunity may be short-lived. Powerful Democratic congressmen have let it be known that when they gain control of Congress, they will rescind the DSHEA legislation. Why they want to remove the right of choice from American citizens and restore total control and power to the FDA and the giant pharmaceutical corporations is beyond my comprehension. Perhaps, they are just uninformed. You may find it advisable to contact your congressional representatives and demand that they keep DSHEA in place. Demand your right of choice—whether to use powerful drugs with their resultant side effects, or herbs and natural foods. Tell them that if they remove this choice from you, you will work to remove them from office at the next election. Then do it!

If the DSHEA legislation is reversed, the FDA will probably require stevia to be removed from all store shelves. It will become illegal for stevia to be sold. Don't let anyone deny you the right to purchase stevia and other herbs and nutritional supplements that are safe for human consumption. I believe FDA-approved drugs cause far more harm and death to an unsuspecting public than do herbs, vitamins, and supplements. The FDA tries to gain support for its agenda by claiming that dietary supplements and herbs are unregulated, thus placing the public at risk. An uniformed, gullible, and gold-hungry media rapidly stirs the pot of deception. The claim is just not true. The FDA and the Federal Trade Commission have all the power they need to remove any and all harmful, fraudulent, mislabeled, or untruthfully advertised products from the market. Herbs, in their natural whole-leaf form, are not drugs. They are foods, to be eaten with wisdom and prudence. Most are no different from tomatoes, carrots, grapes, broccoli, and the dozens of other fruits and vegetables we commonly consume. Some of these foods should be eaten daily, others only during times of need.

Perhaps a copy of this book would enlighten your congressional representatives and senators. If they understood the truth, perhaps they would find the courage to do battle with and reform the FDA, allowing it to once again serve and protect the public from products that really are harmful.

Following the passage of the DSHEA legislation, the FDA immediately set out to nullify and to redefine disease so that virtually all structure-function claims could be construed as disease claims. The approach it is using in this counterattack against herbs seems to be:

1. Locate an individual who uses one or more herbal products who has experienced a harmful episode.

2. Link that reaction to one of those herbal products, whether it was responsible or not.

3. Declare that the herb is harmful and that it and all herbs are dangerous and should be classified as drugs, which must obtain FDA approval before they can be marketed.

4. Do not publicize that the person was also using a prescription drug known for the specific side effect experienced.

For stevia there is more. Declare that it is a natural contraceptive, may cause abnormalities in the male reproductive system, and may cause cancer. These assertions always scare the uninformed. No longer being in absolute control must be difficult to bear.

Stevia Becomes a Nutritional Supplement

Soon after the DSHEA legislation became law in 1995, a multilevel marketing company called Sunrider International notified the FDA of its intent to market stevia as a dietary supplement, following the provisions of the legislation. The FDA had seventy-five days to respond. To deny stevia as a dietary supplement, the FDA now had to prove that it was harmful to consumers, which it did not attempt to do, nor could it have done so. This is because no such proof exists. Perhaps thinking more clearly, the FDA determined that all forms of stevia could be sold as a dietary or nutritional supplement and that structure/function claims must be stated. The label, however, could not describe the product as sweet nor indicate that its function was to enhance the flavor of other foods or beverages. The fire-belching dragon of the artificial sweetener industry was wounded—ever so slightly. The FDA still forbids companies that produce and sell stevia to inform consumers that the herb is sweet. Stevia manufacturers are not permitted to give consumers essential information concerning the herb's sweet taste or its appropriate uses, let alone its health benefits. Some companies marketing stevia "push the envelope," but the regulation issued in 1995 remains in place and is enforced from time to time.

Following the passage of the DSHEA, I returned to Paraguay to again try to persuade the farmers there to grow stevia. They would not believe that stevia could now be sold in the United States. It took me two years to convince them of the potential market, but having already been burned twice, most were not willing to take the financial risk. I "loaned" farmers thousands of dollars to purchase stevia seedlings and to install irrigation systems. They were to pay me back by selling me the leaves at their production cost until the loan had been repaid. Colonel Ramirez, my director of South American operations, however, could never get them to deliver the leaves. Consequently, I could not fill all my orders for stevia leaves and lost tons of sales. The farmers finally admitted the true reason they were not keeping their part of the agreement. Such a demand for stevia leaves had been created and there now were so few stevia farmers that the price of stevia seeds had soared to $100 American per kilo (2.2 pounds). Once a plant flowered, preparatory to producing seeds, its leaves were no longer premium quality, and could not meet my standards.

Other buyers, however, flocked to Paraguay and purchased the poor-quality leaves. These buyers were not knowledgeable about stevia and therefore were not so demanding of quality leaves. I never recovered my loans. The Paraguayan authorities had no interest in helping Americans collect debts from Paraguayans. Another lesson learned. Knowledge, united with experience, brings forth wisdom. By the time quality stevia leaves were again available in abundance, the market in the United States had dried up. Americans now wanted stevia extract (stevioside) products.

The Chinese government had greater foresight than did the officials of the Paraguayan government. The demand for stevia leaves in Asia for the processing of stevioside was great, so China had begun to subsidize its farmers. When the demand for leaves began to grow in the United States, the Chinese flooded the market with very poor quality leaves. Neither the American suppliers nor consumers knew the difference. Many people tasted Chinese stevia and decided it wasn't worth using. They were correct. I tasted those early Chinese leaves sold by one of my competitors. They tasted like dirt. Unfortunately, these consumers lost out on the wonderful health benefits of South American stevia, and many would never again give stevia a try.

At about this time I received a telephone call from a representative of one of America's largest suppliers of herbs. She wanted to sell me stevia leaves from China. I could not restrain my laughter. Upon regaining control of myself, I startled her by suggesting that I would sell her stevia leaves. I explained the difference in quality to her and offered to send her free samples of my Paraguayan leaves so that she could see what stevia really tasted like.

A few days after receiving my Paraguayan leaves, she called me back. She could not believe how sweet they were. She said that she had not understood why stores and manufacturers were buying her company's leaves when they tasted so bad. She placed an order for 1,000 kilos (1 metric ton) of leaves. Unfortunately, that was during the time the Paraguayan farmers were selling seeds in preference to leaves, so I could not fill her order.

Chinese stevia leaves were just not as sweet as South American stevia leaves, and the Chinese farmers still needed to learn to keep their leaves clean and free of dirt and contaminants. Ultimately they did. What the Chinese did right, from the very beginning, was to build processing facilities. They could produce stevioside themselves. It would just take more leaves. Today, most of the stevioside sold in the United States comes from China. Some of it is excellent and some is not. The best bet for consumers is to purchase only brands they feel confident are consistent in quality and reliability. If one brand tastes bad, try another. Quality stevia is worth the search, whatever effort the search requires.

In 1995, following her freshman year at Harvard, my daughter Shannon wanted to provide a service by performing a summer scholastic internship in Paraguay. She had studied Spanish for six years, and wanted to polish her language skills as well as do something worthwhile during the summer. Colonel Ramirez, my director of South American operations, and a descendent of the Guarani Indians, was able to arrange a position for her with the office of Pro-Paraguay. This is the division of the Department of Agriculture that promotes exportation of agricultural products and encourages foreign investments in Paraguay.

Because Shannon was familiar with stevia and the other Paraguayan herbs, she had the opportunity to participate in high-level meetings with "foreigners" who had come to Paraguay to learn about stevia, and perhaps to export it to their own countries. Interestingly, Shannon would go to Beijing the next summer to study and sharpen her Chinese. Harvard would then award her a grant to spend what would have been her senior year at Harvard, in

Beijing. She studied Chinese films and their effects upon the people. She was able to locate and to send to me various books and materials from both of these countries that assisted me in my enterprise.

Even at this late date, Paraguay had no real government program in place to assist its farmers to grow and export stevia leaves, let alone to process them into stevioside. Fifty years had passed since L. A. Gattoni had presented his plan for the commercialization of stevia to the Medical Plants Division of the Instituto Agronomico Nacional de Paraguay, and nothing had been done. As discussed in Chapter 2, Señor Gattoni had advocated the establishment of a stevioside industry in Paraguay as part of the national drive to export products. Shannon participated in a meeting with Frank Folz, a Canadian who was in Asunción to arrange for the exportation of a large volume of leaves. The leaves would be for a project to be undertaken by the government of Canada and Royal Sweet, a privately owned Canadian company that had set up its leaf-processing facility in Monsanto's Chicago NutraSweet factory. South American stevia leaves could be used to produce stevioside until the newly developed Canadian leaves were in sufficient quantity to be commercially viable. Besides, if the Canadian variety could be grown in South America, three to four crops could be harvested each year instead of only one.

It was suggested to Frank that he arrange a meeting with me since my Paraguayan company was recognized as the largest exporter of stevia and other healing herbs to North America.

Frank Folz and I met a few months later in Asunción and discussed the potential of stevia to reduce world hunger and to help eliminate the cultivation of plants used to produce illegal drugs. Having a mutual vision for stevia, we became fast friends. But this really is getting ahead of my story. Suffice it to say that Agriculture Canada is endeavoring to develop its own superior varieties of stevia. The National Research Council of Canada is in the process of developing new methods of processing the leaves and extracting the sweet glycosides. Government officials in Canada have great expectations for stevia. In fact, in 2000 Canadian government officials requested a supply of Wisdom Herbs stevia products. They wanted to display them and to give them away at an international trade show, at the Canadian government's exhibit, to show attendees the potential of stevia.

In 1996, I was invited to participate in a seminar to motivate and train Paraguayan farmers to grow stevia. My next trip to Paraguay was timed to coincide with this program and I was able to attend the initial session. The training was sponsored by the major newspaper in Asunción, *Diario ABC Color,* under the authority of the Ministry of Agriculture and the Ministry of Commerce. Each person completing the course received a certificate, which recognized that my Paraguayan company was a "collaborator," or participant in the project. We were finally on our way, or so I thought. The pitfalls remained numerous and deep but stevia could finally be sold openly in the United States, if it was labeled as a dietary or nutritional supplement. Americans could now experience the incredible healing benefits of stevia.

The war, however, was not over. Only one battle had been won. The FDA was to regroup, marshal its forces, and return to the frontlines with a vengeance. What would this once-noble organization, which I believe had lost the vision of its true purpose for existence, do when it learned that stevia, when ingested as a whole-leaf food, is not only intensely sweet but incredibly healing as well?

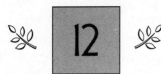

Protector of the Public Interest or Radical Organization?

> "Finally, we should learn a lesson from the NutraSweet ex-
> perience. If a food additive has potential neurological or be-
> havioral effects, it should undergo human clinical testing,
> similar to the process a drug must undergo before it is put
> on the market . . . the food and beverage industry, and their
> various institutes, exert tremendous influence over scientific
> research and investigation. I want to make sure such work is
> genuinely independent."
> —Senator Howard Metzenbaum, testifying at U.S. Senate
> hearing on NutraSweet health and safety concerns,
> November 3, 1987

Unfortunately, many government officials don't learn from the histories of their own organizations or the suffering of the citizens of their countries, nor do they understand their responsibility to prevent health disasters from occurring. When people neglect to learn from history, that history is sure to repeat itself. It is apparent that some government and corporate officials do not learn from the hard lessons of the past, and it appears that they are determined to see those events repeated, if profits can be made. The 1930s to the present have been a time when corporations, sometimes with the approval of the FDA, have put harmful products into the market-place, telling consumers they are the cure for some disease or physical condition. Sometimes these corporations have manipulated the studies, and sometimes they have not fully understood the intricate and delicate workings of the human body. All too often, the long-term consequences have proved disastrous. We can wish that Senator Howard Metzenbaum's hopes for the future are realized, but it does not seem that they will be.

Laws are often passed by Congress and state legislatures with good intentions to protect the public, but based on incomplete or shoddy information. Once in place, these laws are often extremely difficult to reverse, even if they are no longer in the public interest. The status quo is a powerful position. Inertia is difficult to overcome. Even though new information and scientific knowledge come to the fore, there are always powerful forces that work to resist and prevent change.

To complicate matters even further, there are products, such as stevia, and services, such as those offered by holistic or alternative physicians and doctors, that are perfectly safe. The problem is, in my opinion, that well-intentioned people make money, though in small amounts, from these products and services and put a dent, though slight, in the profits of the powerful drug companies and major corporations, which think that all the money to be earned is rightfully theirs.

HEROES OF THE PEOPLE

The Federal Food, Drug and Cosmetic Act of 1938 was absolutely essential for its time. Its purpose was to protect the public from unscrupulous food and drug manufacturers, who, in their quest for profits, were adulterating their products with everything from nondigestible, nonfood ingredients to deadly poisons. Many had little regard for whether their products were clean or contaminated with filth. They cared not whether their products cured or killed the consumer, as long as their bottom line was rising. Under the law of 1906, the FDA routinely lost court cases against such blatant consumer frauds like "strawberry jam" made with pectin, water, grass seed, and very few strawberries.

The 1930s were days of infamy. One notorious incident involved an over-the-counter drug called fluid extract of Jamaica ginger, or Jake for short. Diluted with water, Jake calmed upset stomachs. Drunk straight, however, it packed an alcoholic punch.

This caused it to become popular during Prohibition among people who could not afford good bootleg alcohol. In an effort to make a cheaper Jake and raise the profits, the manufacturer added a chemical that ended up killing some victims and leaving others bed-ridden or crippled for life. Altogether, 35,000 to 50,000 people fell victim.[1]

In those days the FDA was a part of the Department of Agriculture and was permitting arsenic residues, used in pesticides, to remain on vegetables sent to market. Following Franklin Delano Roosevelt's inauguration in 1933, Rexford Tugwell, the new assistant secretary of agriculture, initiated a caustic exchange with Walter Campbell, chief of the FDA. Tugwell objected to a letter about pesticides written by the FDA that recommended balancing farming economics with consumer safety. He wanted to know why the FDA was permitting arsenic residues on vegetables. Campbell, it was reported, stormed into Tugwell's office and explained the FDA's limitations under the 1906 law. Later that day Tugwell set the FDA to work on drafting a new law designed to correct the abuses so prevalent at that time.[2]

The proposed law met with swift opposition from everyone from food and drug manufacturers to newspapers. One journalist, Paul Anderson, wrote in *The Nation*, "The measure frankly challenges the sacred right of freeborn Americans to advertise and sell horse liniment as a remedy for tuberculosis. Which," he added, "stirs men to the very depths of their pocket-books."[3] (While we would hope this was written tongue-in-cheek, it was not so indicated in the FDA report.) With this type of ignorant and selfish opposition, the FDA countered by collecting and exhibiting hundreds of products that had injured or cheated consumers. After being viewed at a Senate hearing, the exhibit was put on public display. No one was sure of President Roosevelt's position on the legislation until his wife, Eleanor, visited the display, with the press at her heels, and dubbed it the "Chamber of Horrors."[4] This vivid description took on a life of its own, and a book of the same name soon followed.

Tugwell's new law, however, was not passed until the next time a poison-laced drug was sold to the American public, which happened in 1937. These years were the genesis of the era of the wonder drugs and no one wanted to hold back progress. German scientists developed sulfamidochrysoidine (Prontosil) and related sulfa drugs that cured bacterial infections such as pneumonia, blood poisoning, and meningitis. One of these was sulfanilamide, which was effective against infections including gonorrhea. Unfortunately, it was difficult to swallow as a tablet and hard to dissolve into a liquid medicine. A chemist of an old and reputable company, S.E. Massengill of Bristol, Tennessee, found a way to dissolve the tablet into a liquid, making it easier for children to swallow. Without any safety testing, the company sent the drug to market, calling it Elixir of Sulfanilamide.[5]

The solvent, diethylene glycol, similar to antifreeze, was a deadly poison. Children who were administered the wonder drug as a medicine for an infected or sore throat suffered intense pain, urine stoppage, vomiting, convulsions, stupor, and death. Heroically, every agent of the FDA scoured the nation, in what the Associated Press called "a nationwide race with death," searching for the remaining pints of the deadly drug. Even though they found and collected 99.2 percent of the elixir of death, 107 unsuspecting people died. Public outrage ensured passage of the Food, Drug, and Cosmetic Act of 1938, with a provision requiring drugs to be cleared for safety before going to market. S.E. Massengill was fined $26,000, the maximum allowed under the law, and the chemist committed suicide.[6]

In the 1930s and 1940s, the FDA was clearly the hero of the safety and well-being of Americans. It was the champion of righteousness. We owe much to the noble souls there who fought the evils of the food and drug industry for our safety. Unfortunately, over the ensuing years, those appointed to administer its balms, and carry out its edicts, seem to have forgotten their endowed purpose.

HERO OF THE PEOPLE OR AGENCY OUT OF CONTROL?

Stevia is one of the most researched agricultural products on earth. It is estimated that more than 1,000 research documents and patents have been published about it. Nearly all the research has been done to prove its safety as a sweetener. It has been assumed that this is where the money is, and this, therefore, has become the primary concern of the pharmaceutical companies and food manufacturers. While wonderful, potential health benefits have also been discovered through this research, they have not been pursued. If a healing benefit is claimed for a food, the FDA will classify that food as a drug. As discussed in Chapter 4, the most recent figures from the drug manufacturers show that it costs from $500 million to $700 million and takes from five to ten years to obtain FDA approval to market a new drug. A whole food cannot be patented, and because others who have not invested time or money in the acquisition of a drug approval can sell the food at a much lower price, there is no incentive either to prove the benefit of or to market the product. In fact, there is a clear disincentive to prove the effectiveness of the product through scientific research. If a food is promoted as being able to help, relieve, mitigate, prevent, or cure a disease, the FDA proclaims that it is an unapproved drug and removes it from the market. The truthfulness of the statement is not a consideration. In direct contrast to this, however, the FDA was willing to take a drug and reclassify it as a sweetener. I must wonder whether this is ignorance, deceit, or an agency that no longer comprehends its mission?

In instances such as this, the FDA functions on the ridiculous premise that it is not necessarily the product itself, or what it does within the body, that determines if the product is a food or a drug, but what is written on the label or in the literature produced by the company for the consumer to read or what is verbally told to the consumer by a seller. If a company that markets carrots were to say that the nutrients in carrots could cure, or even help to prevent, eye disease or degeneration of the eye, the FDA could say that carrots are now a drug. Anyone from that company selling carrots could then be arrested, prosecuted, and even imprisoned for selling an unapproved drug, or for practicing medicine without a license for having prescribed the drug. An honest and informed retailer can be made into a criminal for trying to provide a true benefit to his customers. However, the FDA would not prevent others from selling carrots, as long as they made no health claims. The retailer who teaches and provides true information is punished while competitors who do not inform their customers of the value of the product are allowed to continue in business selling carrots. The consumer is also the loser.

You think this can't happen in America? A few years ago a clerk in a retail health food store in California was asked by a very overweight lady what product she could take to help her lose weight. The clerk was very busy with several customers at the cash register and simply directed her to the book section of the store. She told the lady that there were several books on the subject that she could read. The fat lady was wearing a wire and FDA agents were waiting outside the store, listening to the conversation. The agents stormed into the store and arrested the clerk. Their position was that the clerk had informed the fat lady where to obtain information for a medical condition. The case went to court. Fortunately the judge had more common sense than the FDA agents and acquitted the clerk and the store.

An Abuse of Power

The following story is different in context but reveals a potentially frightening future for Americans. The morning of May 6, 1992, dawned calm and peaceful in Kent, Washington. The office staff at the medical clinic of Jonathan Wright, M.D., a highly respected holistic physician, was preparing for the usual heavy load of patients. At 8:45 there was a loud, intimidating banging on the front door, which then burst open at the same instant that three other clinic doors were kicked in. An estimated two dozen FDA agents and King County police officers rushed into the room from all the doors. Wearing Flak jackets, they leveled their guns at the terrified young female employees. "Freeze! Get your hands up!" they shouted. It was a real SWAT-team-type attack. Only this time it wasn't because the young ladies were violent criminals. They assisted a medical doctor who, in defiance of the decrees of the establishment, practiced holistic medicine.[7]

The women were paralyzed with fear. They would later testify at a hearing that they suffered severe psychological trauma from the experience. One employee would claim physical abuse at the hands of one officer who she said threw her into a chair after he had ripped the phone out of the wall to prevent her from notifying the clinic's attorney of the raid.

The FDA would later claim that guns were not used to terrify the employees. But one employee would testify, "The first agent who broke through the door seemed to have such an adrenaline rush that I really thought he might shoot." Another testified, "The agent told me to get my hands up where he could see them. I said, 'Get serious. This is a doctor's office.' He then moved the gun close to my face and said, 'I said get your hands up.' " An employee from the billing office said, "They just yelled, 'Everyone get your hands up where we can see them.' Their guns were pointed toward us. I was shaking with fear." Perhaps because the officers had turned their identification badges over to hide their names, one brave woman looked at one of the agents and asked, "Does your mother know what you do for a living?"

How could any of these cowardly men ever again look into the eyes of their mothers, wives, or daughters? Is this the way we want innocent medical personnel—or anyone—treated by those in power, just because of a difference in medical philosophy or beliefs?

Dr. Wright arrived about that time but was denied access to his offices. The search and seizure lasted about fourteen hours, during which time neither Dr. Wright, his attorney, nor the owner of the building was allowed to enter and observe the proceedings. The invading agents confiscated the computer hard drive from the clinic's central server along with preservative-free, injectable B-complex vitamins, minerals, and glandular extracts; allergy sensitivity testing equipment; instruction and training manuals; and patient medical records. Everything was loaded into a van and taken away. The press would label the raid the "B-vitamin bust."

In this land of constitutional law, was it impossible for these FDA agents to act like civilized people and simply present the search warrant to Dr. Wright and then calmly examine his clinic for whatever evidence they thought existed there? Although the doctor was not charged with any crime, it took him years to finally get his property, computer hard drive, and medical records back from the FDA. Apparently, the agency feared that his records established its guilt.

The *Seattle Post-Intelligencer* of May 11, 1992, demanded to know why the FDA used "Gestapo-like tactics" in its raid on Dr. Wright's clinic. The FDA quickly took legal measures to have the records of its involvement in the invasion sealed. It wanted no one to know the reason for the raid. Dr. Wright, a licensed physician, had been practicing medicine in the state of Washington for twenty-two years. He had completed his premed studies at Harvard University and had received his medical degree from the University of Michigan. By 1992 he had authored two books and was writing regular columns for *Prevention* and *Let's Live* magazines. He was hardly a criminal to be feared—unless his stethoscope was a deadly weapon.

What, then, was this good doctor's crime? He was, to the best of his extensive medical knowledge, providing the best possible care for his patients, which included effective but all-natural herbs and vitamins. The speculation was that his use over the previous six years of an additive-free B-vitamin complex, derived from adrenal cortex extract and purchased from a manufacturer in Germany, was his crime. The giant American pharmaceutical company Eli Lilly had produced and sold this medication for more than thirty years but had stopped production at the time in favor of a synthetic extract with lower manufacturing costs. Dr. Wright preferred the natural substance rather than the synthetic drug.

It seems evident to me that on May 6, 1992, at least three crimes were committed by the FDA, the agency that is supposed to protect the health and well-being of Americans. First, it invaded an established medical clinic and terrorized the clinic's peaceful employees with the apparent intent, if provoked, to maim and kill the women. (I believe that anyone who breaks through a door with a loaded gun has the intent to shoot at the slightest perceived provocation.) Second, it confiscated private property, without appropriate cause. Third, it denied medical treatment to American citizens, some of whom had traveled more than a thousand miles to see Dr. Wright.

Have Americans become enslaved by the edicts of the FDA and a judicial system that seeks absolute domination of the people rather than their well-being and right of choice? It is incomprehensible that the descendants of a people who went to war to win their freedom from England, then the most powerful nation on earth, would tolerate such actions by an agency of their own government. Where are the Paul Reveres, George Washingtons, John Adamses, Thomas Jeffersons, and Abraham Lincolns of our times?

This is not to say that there are not people in the herbal industry who deserve to be arrested and prosecuted. There are! I believe that there are also medical doctors, pharmacists, pharmaceutical company executives, business executives, government bureaucrats, legal authorities, county and state prosecutors, and law enforcement officers who should be prosecuted for their crimes against innocent people. Those persons in authority who lie, deceive, or cheat customers and consumers, or harm people, should be prosecuted.

For a contrast to the above incident, consider this experience: In early 1989 an FDA agent came into my warehouse to inspect a truckload of herbs that had just arrived from Paraguay. As he was leaving, he noticed a stack of printed papers on a shelf in the warehouse. He quickly put his hand to the side of his face to block his peripheral vision. "If that's literature about your product, I don't even want to see it," he said. "There's nothing you can write about your herbs that we cannot find fault with and prosecute you for." The purpose of his visit, appropriately established by previous appointment, was to inspect the herbs, not to confiscate literature for examination. He was kind to me, and I learned the lesson. To me, this man was a hero.

I have always had excellent relations and experiences with the local agents of the FDA because I have always been honest with them and given them entrance to my offices and warehouse upon their request. They have nearly always treated me as I have treated them. I believe that most local FDA personnel in the various cities of America are honest and honorable men and women, truly trying to protect the health and welfare of American citizens. They have a very difficult job that only increases in difficulty with each passing year as more and more companies introduce harmful foods, beverages, drugs, and dietary supplement products into the market.

These local authorities, however, are required to carry out the directives that come from the Washington, D.C. office, with its revolving door, whether they agree with the directives or not. I suggest that this, for the reasons I have presented, is the seat of the problem. The next chapter will provide insight into what I mean.

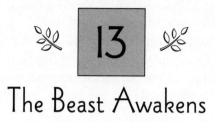

13

The Beast Awakens

"The lip of truth shall be established forever: but a lying tongue is but for a moment."

—Proverbs 12:19

"The wisdom of the prudent is to understand his way: but the folly of fools is deceit."

—Proverbs 14:8

A few weeks after the article about my stevia concentrate, Nectar of HoneyLeaf, appeared in *Vegetarian Times* back in 1985 (see Chapter 2), I was called into the local FDA office. The very apologetic agent informed me that the Washington office had insisted that the local office stop me from importing and selling stevia concentrate. It was obvious that the agent loathed what he was required to do. He told me that there was nothing wrong with the product and that no consumer had complained. He suggested that the makers of NutraSweet wanted stevia out of the market and that they had the influence to get what they wanted. He offered me a deal. If I would just stop importing the stevia concentrate, there would be no record kept of the action against me, nor would the public be notified of an official action against me. There would be nothing to blemish my clean record with the FDA. Since I had never sold more than $200 worth of stevia concentrate in any one month, I readily agreed. After all, what option did I have?

While I could no longer market the stevia concentrate, I continued to bring enough from Paraguay for my own use and especially for that of my youngest daughter. Stevia had performed a miracle for her. I was not about to allow stevia to be taken from her. As I discussed in Chapter 4, since infancy she and Michael had suffered not only from PKU, but also from severe hypoglycemia. The doctors had wanted to remove the pancreases from both of them. I am convinced that stevia saved their pancreases, their brains, and their lives.

In 1988, Oscar Rodes, a native of Brazil who now markets his own brand of Brazilian stevia products, and I traveled together to Maringá, Brazil, to consult with a group that was just finishing construction of a factory to produce stevioside. The group's scientific advisor was Dr. Mauro Alvarez, from the University of Maringá. Dr. Alvarez has done much of the research in South America proving the safety of stevia and stevioside. In addition to meeting with the group, I had the privilege of meeting Dr. Alvarez and discussing his research.

The primary question the group had for me was: "What do we have to do to sell stevioside in the United States?" In preparation for this meeting, I had asked that question of Dr. A. Douglas Kinghorn, whose excellent scientific review titled "Current Status of Stevioside as a Sweetening Agent for Human Use" had been included in Volume 1 of *Economic and Medicinal Plant Research,* published in 1985 by Academic Press. I repeated his reply to me: "It will take at least two million dollars and four to five years of additional research." This group of Brazilian stevia farmers had neither the money nor the time. They had counted on the U.S. market. Not having it available to them would cost them dearly. They would have to concentrate their marketing efforts within Brazil, where stevia had governmental approval. Oscar's problems with the FDA would commence in 1991, when armed federal marshals would raid his warehouse in Arlington, Texas. They would seize his most recent shipment of stevia leaves and stevioside. His difficulties with the FDA would continue for years.

I believe time has proven that aspartame has wrought havoc with the health of consumers. With thousands upon thousands of devastating and documented consumer experiences and medical reports available, only the very foolish refuse to recognize this. For persons who have PKU, ingesting aspartame *will* cause severe brain damage. In the beginning, any product containing aspartame was required to bear a warning notice to people with phenylketonuria. Today, it is difficult to find those statements of warning on products, although a few do carry them. Because two of our own children have PKU, my wife and I are deeply concerned about aspartame and have had to be on constant alert for products containing it. For our children, aspartame is deadly to their brain cells and their quality of life.

What is difficult to comprehend in all of this is that the FDA reported in the October 1988 edition of its own publication, *FDA Consumer*, that 80 percent of all the consumer complaints of adverse reactions it had received since the day the agency came into existence were against aspartame. (As of 2000, that total is 72 to 75 percent of all complaints.) It dismisses these thousands of complaints from consumers, medical doctors, and nutritionists by saying that these people don't know what they are talking about. The FDA approved aspartame as safe, and for some reason, it is prepared to defend its decision regardless of the evidence to the contrary. While the great monster is allowed to roam freely, devouring whom it will, its powerful attendants tie the hands of the weaponless warriors who would engage in competitive battle. Thus, they become easy prey.

I therefore decided to position my product as a "skin refiner," which in truth it is. I had learned from the Guarani how wonderful stevia concentrate is for the health and healing of the skin. Without intending to do so, Searle and the FDA had forced us to learn more about the incredible healing power of stevia. Truly, it is far more than just a sweetener. I learned that the blend of stevia concentrate and Redmond Clay is a remarkable facial mask. Redmond Clay is renowned for its ability to draw toxins from the skin and heal boils, stings, and similar problems. For a recipe for this mask, see page 216.

Perhaps, in reality, this was a blessing in disguise. By promoting stevia concentrate as a facial mask and for the health of the skin, I was to learn even more than the Guarani had taught me about its incredible power to heal the body. As the months passed, delighted consumers called to relate what the product had done, not only for the taste of their food, but also for healing sores and various conditions of their skin—and for lowering or raising their blood sugar. Numerous times I found myself vigorously advising consumers not to eliminate or reduce their insulin until their physician had examined them and instructed them to do so. Stevia concentrate, wearing its dark cosmetic disguise, would remain in the bathrooms and kitchens of America—at least for now.

From the heat that had emanated from the beast and burned my skin, and the juice of the lemon that I had been dealt now stinging my flesh and eyes, I was determined to bake licorice-flavored lemon pie. Besides, I would soon learn that stevia concentrate is wonderful for healing burns—even severe burns. Applied to burns, it stings like fire for a few minutes, but is followed by a wonderful relief of pain, then a remarkably rapid healing. Like the legendary phoenix, stevia would yet rise from the ashes. Let the beast revel in its hot belch of fire. In the end, we will heal our wounds with the very object of its wrath.

Redmond Clay Facial Mask

An oft-used formula for preparing a Redmond Clay facial mask is to mix one teaspoon of Redmond clay with a half-teaspoon of stevia concentrate (dark liquid) and one teaspoon or more of water. Apply the mask to the face and neck, and allow it to dry for ten to fifteen minutes maximum. To remove the mask, moisten it with warm water and wipe it away using a wet cloth. Wash the face several times with warm water to remove all the residue. Blot the face dry and apply a good moisturizer.

ONCE AGAIN THE FDA TAKES ACTION

Following our meetings with the stevia farmers and would-be producers of stevioside in Brazil, Oscar Rodes had the "unmitigated gall" to submit a petition to the FDA to have stevia approved as GRAS. His petition on behalf of his suppliers in Maringá, Brazil, dated December 27, 1988, was ignored. However, the beast and its attendant took notice of this native Brazilian. They would soon be ready to roast and devour another tender morsel in the person of this naïve upstart who dared invade Searle's sweet soil.

By this time, the "big boys" in the tea and herbal beverage industry were also learning about the benefits of stevia. By 1989, Celestial Seasonings, Traditional Medicinals, and numerous other, smaller herb companies, unaware of the fomenting danger, began to add stevia leaves to their herbal teas.[1] After all, theirs was just a nutritious food that had been consumed for centuries. Blending stevia leaves with other herbs was no different from blending lettuce leaves with celery, radishes, cucumbers, carrots, mushrooms, and other nutritious vegetables to produce a delicious-tasting, health-promoting salad. They simply could not claim that their "salad" would improve anyone's health or that the nutrients in it would help the body cure itself of disease. This was a logical assumption for any reasonable mind. (By the way, crushed or powdered South American stevia leaves included in a salad such as this would enhance the flavor and add wonderful nutrition.)

According to estimates, hundreds of tons of stevia leaves were coming into the United States.[2] They were being shipped from several different countries and were being used in various products, to improve flavor and taste. Timothy Moley of the Herb Research Foundation, in an article published by *Delicious Magazine* in March 1994, said that "from 1983 to May 1991 (when the FDA stevia blockade was enacted), millions of Americans drank U.S. manufactured herbal teas containing stevia leaf and reported no adverse reaction."

Even the Lipton Tea Company would petition the FDA to approve stevia leaves as a GRAS ingredient. It wanted to sweeten its teas with the herb. Its petition was ignored. As it had done before, the FDA confiscated the stevia leaves in Celestial Seasonings' warehouse.

Being duly intimidated by this show of force, Celestial Seasonings' executives, according to documents, told the FDA invaders about the other companies using stevia in their products.[3]

How does the FDA account for these invasions and the unwarranted destruction of the legal property of private industry? It admits only to a "trade complaint" filed by an anonymous company. When asked for a copy of the complaint and the name of the company that submitted it, it can no longer find the complaint. There was no statement of a consumer complaint or that anyone had experienced an adverse reaction of any kind to stevia. A "trade complaint" means that someone in the industry had complained about stevia. Note that the targets of such a complaint are never permitted to know the identity of their accuser.[4]

It is difficult to believe that this could happen in the United States of America. Do you understand the magnitude of this situation? The FDA is under the absolute control of one individual, with authority delegated to a few others. I believe these individuals have too much power. There is no court action. There is no public hearing. In the case of stevia, there was no consumer complaint of harm. As one arrogant FDA official told an acquaintance of mine, "If we wanted to make carrots against the law, we could do it." If that doesn't frighten you, it should! The FDA believes it has the power—and the right—to remove any food it chooses from your dinner table, at any time it wants to. You cannot influence its determination nor prevent its action.

The FDA is empowered to enact and enforce its own rules and regulations, which become law. This should cause every American who understands the guarantees afforded under the Constitution of this nation to fear and tremble. Events such as this, in the history of this federal agency, are numerous. Watch your daily newspaper for the many accounts of consumers, medical doctors, and scientists who complain to the FDA concerning drugs and medications that cause serious harm and even death. Regardless of the harm these dangerous substances have caused consumers, the FDA refuses to remove them from the market, while giving great publicity to the remote possibility that herbs might, under some unusual circumstance, cause harm to a few people. Why?

THE GREAT DECEPTION

It is one thing to be confused or to misunderstand, and thus to mislead the people. I believe it is quite another thing to intentionally set out to deceive the very ones you are committed to serve, in order to benefit another.

The FDA has consistently refused to reveal the identity of the company that issued the trade complaint against stevia. How it knew about these manufacturers of herbal teas using stevia remains a mystery. In most cases, stevia was not named on their labels, which listed only a "natural flavoring."

To this day, no complaint of harm or adverse reaction of any kind has been made against stevia by a consumer—not in the United States, nor in Japan, Asia, or South America. No matter how much is consumed, stevia does not cause an increase in weight, blood sugar, cavities, or acne. As Dr. Kinghorn said, "No evidence of adverse reactions due to the ingestion of *S. rebaudiana* extracts of stevioside by humans has appeared in the biomedical literature."[5]

Stevia does not cause a desire for more stevia. In fact, stevia reduces the desire for sweets of all kinds and is a significant aid in weight loss and weight management. Stevia raises the energy level of people with low blood sugar. Clearly, stevia is a safe and healthful sweetener.

On May 17, 1991, the FDA became even more aggressive and issued an "import alert," halting the importation of all stevia and stevia-containing products into the United States. Agents were to seize all stevia at the borders. The import alert was titled "Automatic Detention of Stevia Leaves, Stevioside (Extract of Stevia Leaves) and Food Containing Stevia." This document stated that stevia was an "unsafe food additive" and that its use in foods constituted an "adulteration" of the foods. However, the following statement appeared on the second page of the FDA's import alert:

> Stevia leaves are a native product of Brazil and Paraguay. They have been used throughout history and the extract, Stevioside, has reportedly been approved for use in foods in Brazil and Japan. The product is used in these countries as a table-top sweetener in virtually all food commodities and as a flavor enhancer in such products as teas. The Stevioside is reportedly 250–300 times sweeter than sugar and contributes no calories to the diet.[6]

This statement, written by the FDA to its own agents on an official document, is in direct contradiction to its later statement in denying GRAS status to stevia, declaring that it was "a rare and un-known plant."

The American Herbal Products Association decided to act. On October 21, 1991, its officers began the process of submitting a petition to the FDA. They were told by the FDA to file under the GRAS provision for a food ingredient. Not only was the final two-inch-thick document and the scientific research it contained ignored, but the authorities must have roared with laughter. They now had the AHPA in the catch-22 of the FDA's creation. The AHPA had requested GRAS approval, as instructed by the FDA, for a food ingredient in use prior to 1958 but had included scientific evidence of the safety of stevia. In fact, in September 1993, the Herb Research Foundation wrote a seventeen-page supplement to the original petition, which the AHPA submitted to the FDA. Mark Blumenthal, the executive director of the American Botanical Council and the editor of its quarterly journal, *HerbalGram,* reported:

> The supplement attempted to provide the additional material requested by the FDA, material supporting the use of stevia prior to 1958. The supplement noted that more than 120 scientific and technical articles about stevia were written prior to 1958, only three of them being in lay publications. Even articles written by American scholars and published in journals in the U.S. acknowledged the long-term, safe use of stevia in South America.[7]

This was inappropriate, stated the FDA officials. If filing under the GRAS provision, no scientific evidence is necessary. You must simply prove that the substance was in common use prior to 1958.[8,9] One of the documents that had been submitted was a letter from W. E. Safford, an economic botanist, to the USDA Bureau of Plant Industry, in which he pointed out stevia's commercial value. He incorrectly suggested that the use of stevia had been confined to a small group of Guarani Indians and was unknown by the rest of the world. It was obvious that this was stated as his personal opinion, perhaps to more effectively motivate action toward the commercialization of stevia in the United States. Apparently no one in 1991 had bothered to observe the date of the let-ter—December 18, 1918.

There was a lot of stevia flowing out of Paraguay and Brazil, and being consumed in several countries between 1918 and 1958! But this archaic statement was exactly what the FDA was looking for. It extrapolated this statement to mean that the use of stevia had been confined to a small group of Paraguayan Indians prior to 1958. It refused to file the petition, and yet continuously asked for more re-search, stating that the voluminous scientific documentation al-ready submitted was insufficient.

Besides this, the FDA now had evidence (from one of the scien-tific papers) that stevioside, under controlled laboratory condi-tions, might be harmful, even carcinogenic. This was the cheese in their trap. All one had to do was add a certain solution of mi-croflora produced only in the cecum of a rat along with other toxic chemicals to stevioside and rebaudioside A in a test tube and allow it to incubate for two to six days. The bacteria degraded the stevio-side into a metabolite called steviol, which under these conditions, it was suggested, *might* cause harm to humans. As we have previ-ously learned, the hypothesis could not be proven and, in fact, has never been known to occur, but that didn't matter. Here were sci-entists who said stevioside might somehow be degraded into a sub-stance that *might* be harmful to humans. The fact that millions upon millions of people were consuming stevia or stevioside daily—and without harm—carried no weight. Scientists had man-aged, under manipulated conditions impossible to duplicate within the human anatomy, to produce a carcinogen from stevioside. The public must be protected from carcinogens—even if the carcinogen could be contrived only within the mind and a petri dish.

The fundamental fact that humans do not have a functioning cecum, and that there is no evidence that the human intestinal tract contains the same microorganisms as does that of a rat did not mat-ter. Further, chemists M. Bridel and R. Lavieille had well estab-lished in 1931 that steviosides pass unchanged and unmetabolized though the entire human alimentary canal. They are literally flushed down the toilet, creating the sweetest sewage on earth. No scientific study has ever refuted this finding. These facts totally eliminate the possibility of the conversion process required to create steviol occurring in the human intestine. Apparently that reality just didn't occur to the FDA nor to the scientists involved in the experiment. The only true science to come from this 1980 study, as so succinctly stated by Dr. Mowrey, is that humans are not rats.[10] Well, at least most of us aren't.

It does, however, give a person with a rational mind cause to pause and wonder why this "scientific" group would go to such great lengths to find a potential problem with stevioside.

This brings us to the other evidence of "harm" that had been included in the documents submitted in the petitions to the FDA. As we know, an old study suggested that stevia leaves were a natural contraceptive. In 1968, two researchers set out apparently to prove that stevioside is a natural contraceptive. They wrote that a tribe of natives in Paraguay called the Motto Grosso used stevia as a contraceptive. The results of their primitive and questionable study supposedly established that the treatment was effective for up to two months.

Their hypothesis failed to produce sufficient evidence to allow it to evolve into the category of theory. In addition, for a theory to be established as a scientific fact, the same experiment must *always* produce the same result. Otherwise, the experience reported by the first study is nothing more than an anomaly—a deviation from what would normally be expected. In all the subsequent scientific studies performed to determine the contraceptive properties of stevia, the female rats were naturally impregnated, experienced normal gestation periods, and produced healthy offspring.

Also, all attempts to locate this tribe of Indians have failed. I have asked both the Paraguayan authorities and locals about the existence of this "lost tribe." Dr. D. D. Soejarto searched in vain among the natives living near the origins of stevia. No one has ever heard of them. How can this inconsistency be explained? Were the researchers simply beguiled by a myth? Or was the secret contraceptive tea so effective that the Motto Grosso became extinct, leaving no record of their existence?

However, beyond the fiction of the matter, if stevia leaves were a natural contraceptive, every pharmaceutical company on earth would be clamoring to make and market a totally safe but very high priced stevia-based drug to prevent pregnancy. Some governments of the world would be requiring daily stevia use to reduce the population. Could there be a sweeter, more pleasant way to lower the population of the earth? We should observe, however, that in Japan, China, and Korea, where stevia is in extensive use, no reduction in the birth rate has been reported.

On a personal note, during the last two decades, I have known many women, some of whom were in my employ, who used stevia daily, had normal pregnancies, and produced healthy, bright, and happy babies, bringing great joy to themselves and their stevia-consuming husbands.

ANOTHER GOVERNMENTAL DECEPTION

Once more, the poor Paraguayan farmers were to be deceived by representatives of a foreign government. First, it was by the Japanese authorities. This time it would be by officials of the United States government. In September 1993, following the above described episodes of burning stevia at the stake, Colonel Ramirez, my director of South American operations, and I met with the Paraguayan ambassador to the United States, Juan Esteban Aguirre, in his Washington, D.C., home. I had heard rumors of the following sad tale but I was not fully aware of what had taken place. Around 1989, the U.S. Drug Enforcement Agency (DEA) had met with government officials in Asunción, Paraguay. Their mission had been to persuade the Paraguayan government to stop its farmers from growing marijuana and other illicit drug-producing plants, which were being smuggled into the United States. "What can our farmers grow for a cash crop?" the Paraguayan officials had asked. "They have to be able to earn a living by selling their crops." The reply? "Stevia. They should grow stevia," the DEA agents had answered. "It's an excellent cash crop with a growing market."

The Paraguayan farmers had been reluctant, having been burned once, but they complied with the instructions of their government officials, who had bowed before the pressure of the U.S. government. As soon as their crops were ready for exportation, however, the FDA had placed an embargo on stevia, forbidding its importation into the United States. The farmers lost everything. What could have been crueler and more merciless to these poor farmers, who had just wanted to earn a living and provide for their families?

The total ineptness of it all is difficult to comprehend. One agency of the United States government (the DEA) strongly encourages the production of stevia, virtually insisting that the farmers grow it; at least, that's the way it appeared from the Paraguayan perception of the situation. Then, after the Paraguayan officials and farmers obey the instructions of their "masters," another powerful agency of the U.S. government (the FDA) totally outlaws their crops, literally declaring them to be illegal.

Immediately following my meeting with the ambassador, I met individually with the entire congressional delegation from Arizona and apprised them of the facts in the stevia matter. Each congressman requested that I provide a written review of the situation and a sample letter to the FDA, which some of them transferred to their own official congressional stationary, signed, and sent to the commissioner, David A. Kessler, a medical doctor and attorney. Dr. Kessler had earned his medical degree from Harvard Medical School and his law degree from the University of Chicago. Woe is stevia! But the end is not yet. As was inscribed upon the gold ring worn upon the finger of the wise old king: "And this too shall pass."

Recipes

"Sugar is another dietary disaster ... In addition to causing dental caries [cavities], depressing the immune system, and providing a lot of empty calories that contribute to weight gain, sugar has other detrimental effects, especially for diabetics ... Researcher William Grant ... estimates that sugar intake may account for more than 150,000 premature deaths from heart disease in the U.S. each year.... Consuming large quantities of readily absorbed carbohydrates such as sugar also stresses your body's blood sugar control mechanisms, causing sharp rises in glucose and insulin, followed by precipitous drops. Futhermore, some studies show a link between high sugar intake and chromium loss, which may also contribute to insulin resistance and diabetes. That's a steep price to pay for a food that is devoid of everything but calories—particularly when you eat sugary, processed foods at the expense of whole natural foods."
—Julian Whitaker, *Reversing Diabetes* (Warner Books, 2001)

It is increasingly evident from the vast number of scientific studies available that it is time to eliminate, or at least to significantly reduce, all forms of sugar and artificial sweeteners we take into our bodies. As you have seen in the previous chapters of this book, stevia may well be the very best answer to the sweetener dilemma. But because stevia is so intensely sweet and its flavor is not identical to sugar, you must learn how to cook with its various forms, which range from 30 times sweeter than sugar to 300 times sweeter. Stevia is, however, highly stable in heat, freezing temperatures, and acids. It is compatible with acidic fruits and beverages, including lemons, limes, and oranges, and is delicious on many fruits such as pineapples, strawberries, and blueberries. It is also wonderful with dairy products. Stevia's uses are as varied as your imagination.

Stevia is a natural sweetener and flavor enhancer that not only makes food and drink taste better, but can also nourish the pancreas and help restore and maintain normal blood sugar levels and blood pressure. It can help destroy harmful oral bacteria, reduce cavities, and stop bleeding gums. Where else will you find a sweet herb that in its natural liquid concentrate form is as healing to the skin as it is to the internal function of the body?

To help you begin your own sweet quest for better health and vitality, here are some recipes gleaned from stevia cookbooks available at your local health food store and many bookstores nationwide.

BEVERAGES

Quick Cranberry Punch

Sparkling fresh and alive—sure to jazz up any party

12 ounces frozen unsweetened cran-apple juice concentrate
(thawed)
2 quarts carbonated water (flavored or unflavored)
40 to 50 drops of liquid stevia extract (about ¾ teaspoon) *or* ½
to ¾ teaspoon powdered extract
Slices of oranges and lemons (optional)

Place the unthawed juice, carbonated water, and stevia in a large punch bowl or pitcher just before serving. Serve with round slices of oranges and/or lemons floating on the surface if desired.

Variation: Also excellent with a raspberry juice blend concentrate.
Yield: 8 servings

Recipe reprinted from *Baking with Stevia II: More Recipes for the Sweet Leaf* by Rita DePuydt © 1998 with permission from Sun Coast Enterprises, Oak View, California.

Raspberry Cream

2 cups unsweetened raspberries (fresh or frozen)
1 cup milk (dairy, soy, rice, or almond)
1 teaspoon vanilla
½ teaspoon stevia extract
10 ounces silken tofu
2 tablespoons oil (optional)

Combine raspberries and milk in a blender. Process until smooth. Add vanilla, stevia, tofu, and oil. Blend until creamy. Place in desert glasses. Chill 1 hour or more.

Yield: 4 servings

Recipe reprinted from *Baking with Stevia: Recipes for the Sweet Leaf* by Rita DePuydt © 1997 with permission from Sun Coast Enterprises, Oak View, California.

Strawberry Pina Smoothie

3 cups pineapple juice
2 cups unsweetened strawberries (fresh or frozen)
1 banana (fresh or frozen)
¼ teaspoon stevia extract

Place all ingredients in a blender and process until smooth. Frozen fruit will make the drink thick and creamy.

Yield: 4 servings

Recipe reprinted from *Baking with Stevia: Recipes for the Sweet Leaf* by Rita DePuydt © 1997 with permission from Sun Coast Enterprises, Oak View, California.

BREADS, BISCUITS, AND MUFFINS

Banana Bread

½ cup oil
½ teaspoon stevia extract
1 teaspoon vanilla extract
1 egg (beaten)
½ cup plain yogurt or buttermilk
Juice of ½ lemon
2 ripe bananas (medium-sized)
1 ¾ cups whole wheat pastry flour
¼ cup soy flour
1 teaspoon baking powder
½ teaspoon baking soda
⅛ teaspoon salt
½ cup chopped walnuts (optional)

Preheat oven to 350°. Oil a medium-sized loaf pan.

Combine the oil, stevia, vanilla, and egg in a mixing bowl. Beat until creamy. Beat in the yogurt (or buttermilk) and the lemon juice. Mash bananas in a separate bowl, then fold into the liquid mixture.

Sift the flours, baking powder, baking soda, and salt together. Fold dry ingredients into wet, stirring as little as possible. Mix in the walnuts before flour is completely blended.

Place into medium-sized oiled loaf pan (7 ½ x 3 ½ x 2 ½). Bake 50 minutes to 1 hour until toothpick or fork comes out clean.

Note: For maximum flavor use very ripe bananas.

Yield: 1 loaf

Recipe reprinted from *Baking with Stevia: Recipes for the Sweet Leaf* by Rita DePuydt © 1997 with permission from Sun Coast Enterprises, Oak View, California.

Basic Honey-Wheat Bread

3 ½ cups whole wheat flour
3 tablespoons vital wheat gluten

2 ½ teaspoons active dry yeast
1 teaspoon bread dough enhancer
1 teaspoon salt (optional)
1 ½ cups lukewarm water
2 tablespoons cold-pressed canola or other oil
2 tablespoons honey or molasses
2 teaspoons liquid stevia concentrate

In a large mixing bowl, combine the flour, gluten, yeast, bread dough enhancer, and salt. In a separate bowl, combine the water, oil, honey or molasses, and stevia. Make a well in the dry ingredients, pour in the wet ingredients, and stir with a fork until no longer able. Pour the dough out onto a floured surface and knead until moist but no longer sticky, about 5 minutes. Place in a bread machine pan, place pan in bread machine, and program machine for whole wheat mode.

If the bread touches the bread machine lid during the rising cycle, open the lid and poke the bread with a pin a few times to release some of the air from the "balloon." If you are unable to do this, the very top of the bread will simply remain slightly raw. When the bread is done, just cut the raw part off and discard; the rest of the bread will be fine.

When the machine has completed the baking cycle, remove the bread promptly from the machine and the pan, and place it on a wire rack to cool.

Variation: To make a four-seed bread, add the following ingredients:

½ cup sunflower seeds
½ cup millet
1 tablespoon sesame seeds
1 tablespoon poppy seeds
1 extra tablespoon molasses
1 teaspoon diastatic malt made from sprouted wheat (optional)
1 dash barley malt sweetener

Yield: 1 loaf

Recipe reprinted from *Baking with Stevia: Recipes for the Sweet Leaf* by Rita DePuydt © 1997 with permission from Sun Coast Enterprises, Oak View, California.

Blueberry Muffins

6 ounces pineapple juice
3 tablespoons oil
1 egg (beaten)
½ teaspoon stevia extract
1 teaspoon vanilla extract
½ cup plain yogurt
2 ounces milk
1 cup blueberries (fresh or frozen)
½ cup rolled oats
1 ¾ cups whole wheat pastry flour
1 teaspoon baking soda
½ teaspoon baking powder
¼ teaspoon salt

Preheat oven to 375°. Oil muffin pans.

Soak the oats in the pineapple juice for 10 to 15 minutes in a small bowl.

Beat together the oil, egg, stevia, and vanilla in a mixing bowl. Thin the yogurt with the milk and add to the other liquid ingredients. Beat. Mix in the soaked oats.

Sift together the flour, leavenings, and salt. Fold the dry ingredients into the wet, stirring as little as possible. Fold in the blueberries just before the flour is completely blended.

Spoon batter into muffin pans and bake 25 to 30 minutes.
Yield 12 muffins.

Recipe reprinted from *Baking with Stevia: Recipes for the Sweet Leaf* by Rita DePuydt © 1997 with permission from Sun Coast Enterprises, Oak View, California.

Sweet Butter Biscuits

These biscuits are a delicious breakfast treat, either plain or topped with your favorite fruit spread. And if you like strawberry shortcake, these sweet butter biscuits can serve as the perfect base.

1 ¾ cups all-purpose flour
1 tablespoon double-acting baking powder
½ teaspoon sea salt
⅛ teaspoon white stevia powder
4 tablespoons chilled salted butter
¾ cup cream or milk

Preheat oven to 325°.

Sift together the flour, baking powder, salt, and stevia powder in a large mixing bowl.

Cut the butter into the dry ingredients with a pastry blender or two knives (used scissor fashion) until the mixture is crumbly.

Add the cream, and mix the ingredients with a wooden spoon to form a soft, tacky (not wet) dough.

Turn out the dough onto a lightly floured surface and knead about ten times.

Gently roll out the dough from the center to a ¾-inch thickness.

With a floured 1 ½-inch biscuit cutter, cut straight down into the dough. Place the rounds on an ungreased cookie sheet and bake 10 to 12 minutes, or until golden brown.

Yield: 24 biscuits (1 ½ inch)

Recipe reprinted from *The Stevia Cookbook: Cooking with Nature's Calorie-Free Sweetener* by Ray Sahelian, M.D., and Donna Gates © 1999 with permission from Avery, a division of Penguin-Putnam Publishing Group, New York.

Sweet Corn Mini Muffins

1 cup brown rice baking mix*
1 egg, slightly beaten
¾ cup milk
2 tablespoons coconut oil
1 tablespoon liquid stevia concentrate
1 to 2 cups fresh corn kernels

*Fern's brand is recommended; however, you can substitute this ingredient with 1 cup rice flour, 2 teapoons baking powder, and ½ teaspoon sea salt.

Preheat oven to 400°.

Place the baking mix in a large mixing bowl and set aside. To a blender, add the egg, milk, oil, stevia, and corn, and blend well. Pour this mixture into the baking mix and stir until just mixed. Do not overstir.

Spoon the batter into a lightly oiled or papered mini muffin tin. Fill each cup with a heaping tablespoon of batter and bake for about 12 minutes. When a toothpick inserted into the center of a muffin comes out clean, the muffins are done.

Yield: 24 mini muffins

Recipe reprinted from *The Stevia Cookbook: Cooking with Nature's Calorie-Free Sweetener* by Ray Sahelian, M.D., and Donna Gates © 1999 with permission from Avery, a division of Penguin-Putnam Publishing Group, New York.

Yam Pecan Muffins

1 cup cooked yams (packed)
2 eggs
6 tablespoons oil
2 tablespoons date sugar
⅓ teaspoon powdered stevia extract
¾ teaspoon stevia concentrate
½ teaspoon maple flavoring
1 tablespoon lemon juice

1 cup milk
1 ½ cups whole wheat pastry flour
1 cup unbleached flour
3 tablespoons soy flour
1 teaspoon baking soda
½ teaspoon baking powder
1 teaspoon cinnamon
½ teaspoon nutmeg
¼ teaspoon salt
¾ cup chopped pecans

Preheat oven to 375°. Oil muffin tins.

Cook yams by peeling, cutting, and steaming. Put aside to cool.

In a mixing bowl, beat the eggs into the oil with a wire whisk. Beat in the date sugar, stevia extract, concentrate, and maple flavoring.

In a cup, mix lemon juice and milk. Set aside. While milk is fermenting, sift dry ingredients together and chop the pecans. Beat the soured milk into the egg mixture. Stir in the yams. Break up any large pieces of yam but leave the batter a bit lumpy.

Fold in the dry ingredients. Add the pecans just before the flour is completely mixed in (you may save a small portion of the pecans to sprinkle on the top—lightly press in). Spoon into oiled muffin pans. Bake 25 to 30 minutes. Remove from pan and cool on a rack.

Yield: 12 muffins

CAKES AND PIES

Carrot Cake

½ cup unsweetened coconut
6 ounces crushed pineapple with juice (8-ounce can)
1 teaspoon stevia extract
2 to 3 tablespoons Fruitsource or date sugar
½ cup butter or margarine (softened)
2 eggs (beaten)
⅓ cup yogurt
¼ cup milk
1 teaspoon vanilla extract
½ teaspoon maple flavoring
½ cup chopped walnuts
2 cups grated carrots
1 cup whole wheat pastry flour
1 cup unbleached white flour
2 tablespoons soy flour
2 teaspoons baking powder
1 teaspoon baking soda
1 ½ teaspoons cinnamon
1/4 teaspoon salt
Cream cheese frosting

Preheat oven to 350°. Oil an 8-inch spring-release pan or a 10 x 6-inch cake pan.

Soak the coconut in the pineapple and juice. Use all the juice from an 8-ounce can of pineapple but only 6 ounces of the pineapple. Set aside.

Soften and cream the butter (or margarine) in a large mixing bowl. Cream in the stevia and the Fruitsource (or date sugar). Gradually cream in the beaten eggs (they need to be at room temperature). Don't worry if the butter separates.

Thin the yogurt with the milk and add to the butter. Mix in the vanilla and maple flavoring. Stir in the walnuts, soaked coconut, pineapple, and carrots.

Sift the flours, leavenings, cinnamon, and salt together twice in a separate bowl.

Fold the sifted dry ingredients into the wet, stirring just until blended. Batter will be stiff.

Spoon batter into cake pan and bake for 1 hour. Cool in the pan. Release the pan and top with cream cheese frosting.

Yield: 8-inch cake

Recipe reprinted from *Baking with Stevia: Recipes for the Sweet Leaf* by Rita DePuydt © 1997 with permission from Sun Coast Enterprises, Oak View, California.

Coconut Banana Cream Pie

Single pie crust, prepared
4 chopped dates
1 ½ cups soy milk
½ cup unsweetened coconut
1 ⅓ cups water
½ teaspoon stevia extract
1 teaspoon vanilla extract
3 tablespoons arrowroot powder
1 cup tofu whipped cream
1 ½ tablespoons agar-agar (or 1 package gelatin)
2 medium bananas

Grind the chopped dates in a blender with ½ cup of the milk until fairly smooth. Add the coconut and 1 cup of water. Grind and process until creamy. Blend in the rest of the milk. Add the stevia, vanilla, and the arrowroot powder and blend. Note: May use a food processor.

Pour the well-blended mixture into a pan and cook while stirring over medium-low heat until thick. Simmer on low heat for 3 to 5 minutes more, stirring occasionally but gently.

Place the tofu whipped cream in a blender. Place the agar-agar and ⅓ cup water in a small sauce pan. Bring to a boil, then simmer 3 to 4 minutes until dissolved. Add the dissolved agar-agar to the tofu whipped cream in the blender and mix. Fold into the pudding.

Layer sliced bananas in the bottom of the cooled pre-baked pie shell. If preferred, half of the bananas may be mashed and folded into the pudding. Pour pudding over bananas in the pie shell.

Dust top of pie with shredded coconut. Chill in the refrigerator at least 2 hours.

Note: If you don't have any agar-agar (or gelatin), just use an extra tablespoon or two of arrowroot powder. However, the agar gives a creamier, lighter filling with better shape.

Yield: 8- or 9-inch pie

Recipe reprinted from *Baking with Stevia: Recipes for the Sweet Leaf* by Rita DePuydt © 1997 with permission from Sun Coast Enterprises, Oak View, California.

Pumpkin Pie

4 cups cooked, mashed butternut squash
1 teaspoon pumpkin spice
1 tablespoon vanilla flavoring
1/4 teaspoon white stevia powder
Pinch sea salt
9-inch pie crust, prepared

Place all of the filling ingredients in a blender or food processor and blend until smooth and well-combined.

Pour the filling mixture into the crust and refrigerate for at least 1 hour.

Serve chilled or at room temperature, either plain or topped with a dollop of whipped cream.

Yield: 9-inch pie

Recipe reprinted from *The Stevia Cookbook: Cooking with Nature's Calorie-Free Sweetener* by Ray Sahelian, M.D., and Donna Gates © 1999 with permission from Avery, a division of Penguin-Putnam Publishing Group, New York.

COOKIES AND DESSERTS

Apple Bars

Very moist, chewy squares. Lightly spiced.

¼ cup butter, softened
3 tablespoons vegetable oil
¾ teaspoon stevia extract powder
1 teaspoon vanilla extract
2 eggs
1 cup plus 1 tablespoon whole wheat pastry flour
¼ teaspoon salt
1 teaspoon cinnamon
⅛ teaspoon nutmeg
1 teaspoon baking powder
1 ⅓ cups grated apples
⅓ cup chopped walnuts

In a medium bowl beat together butter, oil, stevia, vanilla extract, and eggs. Sift or stir together dry ingredients and stir into the butter mixture using a mixing spoon. Add apples and nuts and mix in. Batter will be stiff. Turn into oiled and floured 9-inch square baking dish. Cook at 350° for 35 to 37 minutes in a preheated oven. Cool about 10 minutes and then cut into bars. Serve warm or cooled. Refrigerate leftovers.

Yield: 16 bars

Fudgy Brownies

Fudge type moist carob cookie bars.

1 cup unsweetened carob chips
½ cup butter
½ cup plus 1 tablespoon whole wheat pastry flour
1 teaspoon stevia extract powder *or* 3 teaspoons green stevia
   powder
¼ teaspoon cinnamon
Shake each of nutmeg and allspice
1 teaspoon baking soda
2 eggs lightly beaten
2 teaspoons vanilla extract
½ teaspoon black walnut flavoring
4 tablespoons plain low fat yogurt *or* 3 tablespoons soymilk
½ cup rolled oats, lightly chopped in a blender
½ cup chopped walnuts

Oil a 9-inch square baking pan. Place chips and butter in a double boiler pan over boiling water. Turn heat to medium-low. Stir occasionally and heat to melt most of the chips.

While chips are melting, mix flour, stevia, spices, and baking soda in a medium bowl. In a second bowl, combine eggs, extracts, and yogurt. Add chopped oats and set aside 15 minutes.

Remove carob mixture from heat. Quickly stir in dry ingredients and egg mixture. Turn into the prepared pan. Sprinkle walnuts over the surface and press in lightly with a spatula.

Bake in a 325° preheated oven for 16 to 19 minutes. Brownies should pull away from the sides of the pan. Do not overcook. Cool on a wire rack. Cut into squares.

Variation: For a drier bar, add an additional 2 tablespoons flour.
Yield: 16 brownies

Recipe reprinted from *Stevia Sweet Recipes: Sugar-Free—Naturally!* (Second Edition) © 1999 by Jeffrey Goettemoeller with permission from Vital Health Publishing, Ridgefield, CT. This is a book of nearly 200 tasty recipes of all kinds using stevia powder and extract as the sweetener.

Granola Energy Bars

2 teaspoons powdered stevia leaf
2 cups granola (use your favorite—if it has chopped nuts and dried fruit, all the better)
⅓ cup tahini, cashew, or almond butter
2 tablespoons oil
⅓ cup apple butter
1 tablespoon liquid Fruitsource or honey
⅓ teaspoon stevia extract
1 teaspoon vanilla

Preheat oven to 375°. Oil a 5 x 9-inch baking dish.

Mix the powdered stevia leaf into the granola in a large mixing bowl.

In a small bowl mix the nut butter and the oil together. Add the apple butter, Fruitsource (or honey), stevia extract, and vanilla. Gently stir this mixture into the granola.

Press the batter firmly and evenly into the baking dish. Bake 18 to 20 minutes. Cool completely before cutting.

Variation: Add 1 heaping tablespoon protein powder to batter.
Yield: 15 bars

Recipe reprinted from *Baking with Stevia II: More Recipes for the Sweet Leaf* by Rita DePuydt © 1998 with permission from Sun Coast Enterprises, Oak View, California.

Maple Nut Ice Cream

2 cups half and half
1 cup milk
2 tablespoons maple syrup
½ teaspoon maple flavoring
¾ teaspoon powdered stevia extract
½ cup chopped walnuts

Blend all the ingredients together except the nuts. Pour into an ice cream machine and process. Add the chopped walnuts about halfway into the freezing process. Nuts should be no bigger in size than a chocolate chip.

Yield: About 1 quart

Recipe reprinted from *Baking with Stevia II: More Recipes for the Sweet Leaf* by Rita DePuydt © 1998 with permission from Sun Coast Enterprises, Oak View, California.

SALAD

Waldorf Salad

7 to 8 Red Delicious apples, unpeeled, cored, and cut into ½-inch cubes (about 4 cups)
1 cup raisins
1 cup coarsely chopped pecans
1 cup shredded carrot
¼ cup plus 2 tablespoons shredded unsweetened coconut

Dressing

1 x 1-inch piece fresh ginger
1 cup mayonnaise
½ cup lemon juice
⅛ teaspoon white stevia powder

Grate the ginger. Using your hands, squeeze its juice into a small bowl. Add the mayonnaise, lemon juice, and stevia. Mix well.

In a salad bowl, combine the apples, raisins, pecans, carrot, and coconut. Add the dressing and toss well.

Cover the bowl and chill in the refrigerator for several hours before serving.

Yield: 4 to 6 servings

Recipe reprinted from *The Stevia Cookbook: Cooking with Nature's Calorie-Free Sweetener* by Ray Sahelian, M.D., and Donna Gates © 1999 with permission from Avery, a division of Penguin-Putnam Publishing Group, New York.

TOPPING

Maple Syrup

¾ cup filtered water
2 tablespoons plus 2 teaspoons vegetable glycerine*
2 teaspoons nonalcoholic maple flavoring
⅛ teaspoon white stevia powder

* Derived from coconut oil, vegetable glycerine is a sweet-tasting thickener. It is available in most health food stores.

Combine all of the ingredients in a small bowl and mix well. You can also place the ingredients in a clean glass jar, cover with a lid, and shake thoroughly.

Warm the mixture in a small pan before drizzling it over pancakes, waffles, or hot cereal.

Yield: About ¾ cup

Recipe reprinted from *The Stevia Cookbook: Cooking with Nature's Calorie-Free Sweetener* by Ray Sahelian, M.D., and Donna Gates © 1999 with permission from Avery, a division of Penguin-Putnam Publishing Group, New York.

CONCLUSION

"All the progress the world has made is owed to the teacher, who sees the vision of the future, perseveres with courage, shares the vision with its promise for a better world, and labors to bring it to pass."
—Havana May, mother of Jim May

The years of my involvement with stevia since 1982 have been filled with heart-wrenching, mind-boggling turmoil ranging from elation to despair and back. There was my initial vision for the future, followed by the financial havoc that came from my investing everything in a business that soon appeared doomed to failure. There were my constant fears that the FDA would totally outlaw and confiscate my stevia, as well as my other Paraguayan herbal products because they contained stevia, or initiate my arrest for simply giving the public too much correct information by spoken word or pen. There were my fears of arrest in Paraguay for photographing the wrong street or building, and the violent military coups that changed the government, its policies, and its agenda. There were always the weeks, months, and years of hard work, long hours, and separation from my family. I was constantly walking to the edge of the light, not knowing what lay ahead in the cloudy mists of darkness. Was it a precipice, a tornado, or calm and tranquil waters? Hope and faith kept me moving ever forward.

For the most part, the fear and trepidation have passed, although not entirely. The FDA has lightened up somewhat, even though its regulations are still in force. It is more likely to initiate proceedings against a company with a warning letter than with armed storm troopers. Besides, it's a different era now. Americans are learning about stevia, and it is being sold everywhere. Various forms and blends of stevia are sold in health food stores, major regional and national grocery chain stores, and drugstores, as well as on several internet Web sites. National magazines are carrying favorable articles about the health benefits of stevia. Holistically minded doctors, health practitioners, nutritionists, and dietitians are recommending it to patients and clients. Several stevia cookbooks have been published containing hundreds of recipes for using stevia in virtually every type of food imaginable that requires sweetening. Not only is stevia now used freely in the kitchens of America, but it is making its way into delis, cafés, and restaurants. Single-serving packets may soon be found on hospital food trays and in the rooms of hotels. There is growing interest in creating energizing nutritional-supplement beverages with stevia, included for its health benefits rather than its sweetening power.

Yesterday I had a most pleasant and rewarding experience. I was receiving a checkup from my family doctor. In answer to a question, I mentioned that I was just making the final corrections to this book. He had never heard of stevia and wanted to know more. We talked about stevia for about twenty to twenty-five minutes— which reveals his keen interest, considering the hectic schedule of this very busy family physician. He was fascinated, then *told me* about the dangers of aspartame and said that he would like a safe sweetener for his family, staff, and patients. I offered to send him some product samples and scientific literature, which he gratefully accepted. He said that after reading the materials and trying the samples, if he found stevia to be all that I had said, he would be willing to recommend it to his patients, especially the ones with diabetes or a weight problem.

Could it be that stevia's day has finally arrived and that Americans and Europeans will demand and use it as their preferred sweetener? If so, I predict a significant improvement in their health, vitality, and well-being, as well as a meaningful reduction in the time and money they spend on their medical care.

I began this magnificent quest not as a salesman, as some may have supposed, but as a teacher. The salesman is motivated by gain. The teacher is motivated by a genuine concern for and sincere valuing of other people, including their physical health and well-being as well as their acquisition of knowledge and wisdom. I understood the health-improving potential of stevia and set out to change the paradigm of my generation—and thus, of generations to come.

As knowledge about stevia gently distills upon the nation, can you imagine the inner joy I feel as the one who originally introduced stevia to America as a commercial product and who, since 1982, has faced head-on the wrath of stevia's opponents and the obstacles they set up? It has been both my joy and privilege to march in the front ranks and to lead in the effort to educate Americans about stevia through the spoken and written word.

During the first quarter of 2003, I was invited to address the Stevia Council, an association of stevia farmers and interested citizens, at a meeting held in the *Diario ABC Color* building in Asunción, Paraguay. *Diario ABC Color* is the major newspaper in Asunción. The group wanted to know the current status of stevia in America and its potential for the future. Steve and I showed them several of the stevia products that we make and market in North America and shared our vision. They were ecstatic. Once again, they began to see the sweet possibilities for this native Paraguayan plant. Their once-waning enthusiasm was renewed.

The newly elected president of Paraguay, Nicanor Duarte Frutos, took office August 15, 2003. He has caught the vision of stevia and the agricultural and industrial potential it holds for his country and its people. He has appointed Antonio Ibañez as the new minister of agriculture, and Señor Ibañez has in turn appointed my good friend Peter Matias Gibert, an executive of *Diario ABC Color*, Paraguay's most important newspaper, to head up the Stevia Project and to investigate what can be done to move the cause of stevia forward. The Ministry of Health is interested in promoting stevia because of its beneficial properties for diabetics.

Señor Gibert has requested input from all interested parties in Paraguay for the development of a National Stevia Plan. Several working committees have been formed, and my Paraguayan company is participating. President-elect Frutos sent a delegation to Washington D.C., to meet with officials of the International Monetary Fund, who, it is said, promised $250 million to help the new government with its development plans for Paraguay. Hopefully, some of those funds will be used for the National Stevia Plan. While this is a beginning, there is still much to be accomplished.

Before stevia can have a positive impact upon the economic future of Paraguay and other South American countries, its worldwide consumption must increase dramatically. New uses, backed by science, must be found for the leaves of this incredible plant. The political powers that block stevia from providing consumers with its health benefits and its great potential as the safest sweetener on earth must stand aside. We will see all of this unfold over the next few years.

However, the end of the story is not yet for "the miracle of stevia." Another triumph waits, perhaps just beyond the horizon. Stevia has the potential to offer another vital blessing to mankind. My friend and fellow stevia enthusiast Dr Frank Folz, working with officials of the government of Bolivia and poor Bolivian farmers during the first half of the decade of the 1990s, proved that stevia is a viable alternative crop to coca. Following years of research and experimentation in Bolivia, Dr. Folz wrote:

> Stevia is seen in all sectors of Bolivian society as a realistic economic alternative for, but not limited to, coca plant production. Bolivia is the world's second largest producer of coca leaves, the raw material for the cocaine drug. The Bolivian government is under heavy international pressure to reduce the number of hectares under coca cultivation. However, the replacement products available to date such as pineapple, heart of palms, bananas, etc. do not produce sufficient return to dissuade peasant farmers from growing coca. The viability study demonstrates stevia's potential to compete with coca in the Bolivian market place.[1]

If and when the Food and Drug Administration, the Drug Enforcement Agency, and other government agencies of the United States and South America get their priorities straight and coordinate their efforts, stevia has the potential to significantly reduce drug traffic throughout the world. This small, innocuous plant, consumed by the people of South America for at least 1,500 years, by the people of the Orient for more than 30 years, and by people in the United States for a decade, has the potential to provide numerous miracles of improved health for mankind. It can also reduce the devastating health problems and horrific crimes caused by the use of illicit drugs and the trafficking thereof. Logically, this in turn could reduce the necessity for the continuing covert actions of U.S. military personnel in drug-producing countries and the number of lives lost in such enforcement tactics.

How can you help? Use stevia. Ask your favorite stores to stock it in its several consumer forms. Try it for the varying purposes with which you are now familiar. When the demand for stevia increases sufficiently, the powers that be may awaken and remove the obstacles. When stevia begins to fulfill its destiny as the safest, most-problem-free sweetener on earth, appearing in food and beverages everywhere, it will also provide a fair income for the poor farmers of Third World countries, who will no longer need to grow drug-producing plants. May that day dawn soon.

APPENDIX A

Approximate Stevia Sweetness Equivalents

Stevia	Sugar
⅓ to ½ teaspoon white extract powder	1 cup sugar
1 teaspoon clear liquid	1 cup sugar
1 tablespoon dark liquid concentrate (water-based)	1 cup sugar
1 ½ to 2 tablespoons ground leaf	1 cup sugar
1 ½ to 2 tablespoons SteviaPlus powder	1 cup sugar
18 to 24 SteviaPlus packets	1 cup sugar
2 teaspoons dark liquid concentrate (water-based)	1 cup brown sugar

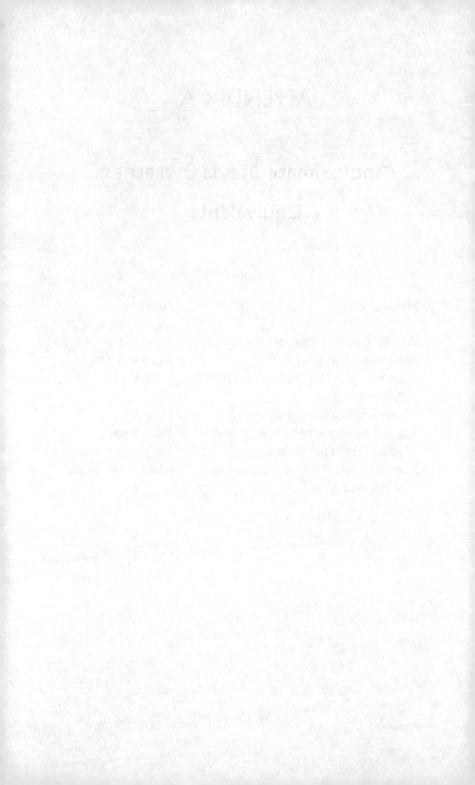

APPENDIX B

Cookbooks

Several excellent cookbooks are available to help you get started replacing sugar and other sweeteners with stevia. Some of them are:

DePuydt, Rita. *Baking with Stevia,* Volume I. Oak View, CA: Sun Coast Enterprises, 1997. Includes 52 recipes.

DePuydt, Rita. *Baking with Stevia,* Volume II. Oak View, CA: Sun Coast Enterprises, 1998. Includes 60 recipes.

Gittleman, Ann Louise. *The Fat Flush Cookbook.* New York: McGraw-Hill, 2002. Includes more than 200 recipes, many of which utilize stevia.

Goettemoeller, Jeffrey. *Stevia Sweet Recipes: Sugar-Free—Naturally!* Ridgefield, CT: Vital Health Publishing, 1999. Includes more than 165 recipes.

Richard, David. *Stevia Rebaudiana: Nature's Sweet Secret,* Third Edition. Ridgefield, CT: Vital Health Publishing, 1999. Includes more than a dozen recipes.

Sahelian, Ray, and Donna Gates. *The Stevia Cookbook: Cooking with Nature's Calorie-Free Sweetener.* Garden City Park, NY: Avery Publishing Group, 1999. Includes more than 100 recipes.

RESOURCE LIST

Stevia products are available in many health food stores, super-markets, and pharmacies. If your local store does not carry stevia products, ask the manager to order them. Stevia products are also available online and by calling the manufacturer or distributor. The major manufacturers and suppliers of consumer stevia products are listed below.

Wisdom Herbs
2546 West Birchwood Avenue
Suite 104
Mesa, AZ 85202
Toll-free: (800) 899-9908
Website: www.wisdomherbs.com, www.steviaplus.com
E-mail: wisdom@wisdomherbs.com
Manufactures and markets SweetLeaf and Wisdom of the Ancients brands of stevia products.

NATURAL FOODS INDUSTRY

Body Ecology
2103 North Decatur Road
Suite 224
Decatur, GA 30033
Telephone: (770) 385-6333
Website: bodyecologydiet.com
E-mail: orders@bodyecologydiet.com
Distributes a clear liquid stevia extract.

Nature's Way
10 Mountain Springs Parkway
Springville, UT 84663
Telephone: (801) 489-1500
Website: naturesway.com
Distributes a stevia concentrate.

NOW Foods
550 Mitchell
Glendale Heights, IL 60139
Telephone: (708) 545-9000
Website: nowfoods.com
Distributes a stevia extract powder and a blended stevioside product.

NuNaturals
2220 West 2nd Avenue #1
Eugene, OR 97402
Telephone: (541) 344-9785
Toll-free: (800) 753-4372
Website: nunaturals.com
Distributes a clear liquid stevia extract.

Planetary Formulas
P.O. Box 533
Soquel, CA 95073
Telephone: (831) 438-1700
Toll-free: (800) 606-6226
Website: planetaryformulas.com
E-mail: ranaw@thresholdent.com
Distributes a stevia concentrate.

Stevita Company, Inc
7650 U.S. Highway 287 #100
Arlington, TX 76001
Telephone: (817) 483-0044
Website: www.stevitastevia.com
E-mail: mail@stevitastevia.com
Distributes several blended stevioside products.

NETWORK MARKETING COMPANIES

Amazon Herb Company
1002 Jupiter Park Lane
Jupiter, FL 33458
Telephone: (561) 575-7663
Website: www.rainforestbio.com/sm/
E-mail: sm@rainforestbio.com
Distributes a clear liquid stevia extract.

Empower Net
1220 North Spencer
Mesa, AZ 85203
Telephone: (480) 649-9664
Website: www.empowernet.com
Distributes a stevia concentrate and stevia tea.

Lowcarbmall.com
1310 East Broadway
Suite 130
Tempe, AZ 85282
Telephone: (480) 517-1555
Distributes all forms of stevia products.

Optimal Health Systems
49 South Sycamore
Suite 3
Mesa, AZ 85202
Telephone: (480) 890-2221
Website: optimalhealthsystems.com
E-mail: info@optimalhealthsystems.com
Distributes a blended stevioside product.

Sunrider International
1625 Ablone Avenue
Torrance, CA 90501
Telephone: (310) 781-3808
Website: www.sunrider.com
E-mail: info@sunrider.com
Distributes a stevia concentrate.

Young Living Essential Oils
250 South Main Street
Payson, UT 84651
Telephone: (801) 418-8900
Distributes a stevia extract, a stevia concentrate, and a blended stevioside product.

NOTES

INTRODUCTION

1. Toufexis, Anastasia, "The New Scoop on Vitamins," *Time,* April 6, 1992, 54–59.

2. *JAMA,* 287, 23:3116–26, 2002.

3. *JAMA,* 287, 23:3223–29, 2002.

CHAPTER 2

1. Report prepared in 1991 for James A. May under the direction of Dr. José Martino Vargas, General Director of the National Institute of Technology and Standardization. Written by Dr. Laura Fracchia, Instrumental Analysis Laboratory, and Dr. Miguel González Moreira, Director of the Central Analysis Laboratory. Document on file.

2. Gosling, C., "Ca á-êhê or Azúca-ca," Kew Bulletin, 173–74.

3. Written statement obtained from the Ministry of Agriculture and Livestock, General Planning Division, under the seal of the Republic of Paraguay, 1993. Document on file.

4. Bell, F., "Stevioside: A Unique Sweetening Agent," *Chemistry and Industry,* 1954, 897–98.

5. Ibid.

6. Bertoni, M. S., "La Estivina y la Rebaudiana, Nuevas Substancias Edulcorantes" (Stevina and Rebaudiana, New Sweetening Substances), Anales Cientificos Paraguayos, 6 De Botánica, Serie II, Num. 2, 1918.

7. Bridel, M., and Lavieille, R., *Journal of Pharmaceutical Chemistry,* 1931, 14, 99.

8. Pomaret, M., and Lavieille, R., *Bulletin of the Society of Chemical Biology,* 1931, 13, 1248.

9. Phillips, K. C., "Stevia: Steps in Developing a New Sweetener,"

in Grenby, T. H. (Ed.), *Developments in Sweeteners—3,* Elsevier Applied Science, London, 1987.

10. "History of the Sugarbeet," *Sugar,* www.sugarproducer.com.

11. Report prepared in 1991 for James A. May under the direction of Dr. José Martino Vargas, General Director of the National Institute of Technology and Standardization. Written by Dr. Laura Fracchia, Instrumental Analysis Laboratory, and Dr. Miguel González Moreira, Director of the Central Analysis Laboratory. Document on file.

12. Fujita, Hideo, and Edahiro, Tomoyoshi, "Safety and Utilization of Stevia Sweetener," Ikeda Tohka. Co., Ltd., 65, 1979.

13. Bridel and Lavieille, op. cit.

14. Shock, Clinton C., "Experimental Cultivation of Rebaudi's Stevia in California," *Agronomy Progress Report No. 122,* Agricultural Experiment Station, University of California, Davis, April 1982.

15. Shock, Clinton C., "Rebaudi's Stevia: Natural Noncaloric Sweeteners," California Agriculture, 1–5, September-October 1982.

16. Phillips, op. cit.

CHAPTER 3

1. Airola, Pavvo, *How to Get Well,* Health Plus Publishers, Phoenix, AZ, 1988.

2. Kinghorn, A. D., and Soejarto, D. D., "Current Status of Stevioside as a Sweetening Agent for Human Use," *Economic and Medicinal Plant Research,* Vol. 1, 1985, 6–9.

3. Richard, David, *Stevia Rebaudiana:* Nature's *Sweet* Secret, Blue Heron Press, Bloomingdale, IL, 1996, 19.

4. Kinghorn, A. D., Ph.D., "Food Ingredient Safety Review: *Stevia Rebaudiana* Leaves," University of Illinois at Chicago, 1992, 36.

5. Rajbhandari, A., and Roberts, M. F., "The Flavonoids of *Stevia rebaudiana,"* Journal of Natural Products, 1983, 46,194–95.

6. Kinghorn and Soejarto, op. cit., 37.

7. Liebman, Bonnie, and Hurley, Jayne, "Vegetables, Vitamin K Weighs In," *Nutrition Action HealthLetter,* Center for Science in the Public Interest, Washington, D.C., July/August 2002, 13–15.

CHAPTER 4

1. Sahelian, Ray, M.D., and Gates, Donna, *The Stevia Cookbook,* Avery Publishing Group, Garden City Park, NY, 1999, 45–46.

2. Whitaker, Julian, M.D., *Reversing Diabetes,* Warner Books, A Time Warner Company, New York, 2001, 253–54.

3. McKeith, Gillian, *Living Food for Health: 12 Natural Superfoods to Transform Your Health,* Judy Piatkus Limited, London, 2000, 125–26.

4. Ibid., 130.

CHAPTER 6

1. Pearson, Durk, and Shaw, Sandy, *Life Extension, A Practical Scientific Approach,* Warner Books, Inc., New York, 1982, 292.

2. Ornstein, Robert, and Sobel, David, *The Healing Brain,* Simon and Schuster, New York, 1987, 47.

3. Genesis, Chapter 41, Old Testament, King James Version.

4. Gittleman, op. cit., 172.

5. Cabot, Sandra, M.D., Press release provided by Betty Martini, Mission Possible International, at http://www.dorway.com.

6. Gittleman, op. cit., 13–15.

7. Page, Linda, N.D., Ph.D., "Discover Your Weight Loss Blocker," *Total Health for Longevity Magazine,* Vol. 24, No. 3, 48.

8. Conyers, Georgia, at http://www.newtonlabs.net, and http://www.dorway.com.

9. Remington, Dennis, M.D.; Fisher, Garth, Ph.D.; and Parent, Edward, Ph.D., *How to Lower Your Fat Thermostat,* Vitality House International, Inc., Provo, UT, 1987, 24.

10. Ibid. 1–2.

11. Ibid. 1–4.

12. Gittleman, op. cit., 6–7, 29–30.

CHAPTER 7

1. Kinghorn, A. D., Ph.D., "Food Ingredient Safety Review: *Stevia rebaudiana* Leaves," University of Illinois at Chicago, 1992.

2. Kinghorn, A. D., Ph.D. (Ed.), *Stevia: The Genus Stevia,* Taylor and Francis, London, 2002, ix.

3. Planas, G. M. and Kuc, J., "Contraceptive Properties of *Stevia Rebaudiana,*" *Science,* 1968. 162,1,007.

4. Kinghorn, 1992, op. cit.

5. Kinghorn, A. D. and Soejarto, D. D., "Current Status of Stevioside as a Sweetening Agent for Human Use," *Economic and Medicinal Plant Research,* Vol. 1, 1985, 1–52.

6. Soejarto, D. D.; Compadre, C. M.; Medon, P. J.; Kamath, S. K.; and Kinghorn, A. D., *Economic Botany* 1983, 37, 71.

7. Moreno, A. R., *La Medicina en El Paraguay Natural,* 1771.

8. Anaia, P. N., *Botanica Medica Americana—Los Herbarios de Las Misiones de Paraguay,* Administracio de la Biblioteca, Buenos Aries, 1898.

9. Rodrigues, P. M., *Plantas Medicinales del Paraguay,* Imp. La Mundial, Asunción, 1915.

10. *Planta Medicinales usadas por el vulgo en el Paraguay,* Imp. Nacional Paraguay, 1924.

11. Bertoni, M. S., *La Medicina Guarani,* Y Edicion Ex-Sylvis, Paraguay, 1927.

12. Michalowski, M., *Plantas Medicinales del Paraguay,* Ministerio de Agricultura y Ganaderia, Asuncion, 1955.

13. Steward, J. H. (Ed.), *Handbook of the South American Indians,* Smithsonian Institution, Bureau of Ethnology, Washington, D.C. 1946.

14. Strauss, L., *Handbook of the South American Indians,* Vol. 6, J. H. Steward (Ed.), Smithsonian Institution, Bureau of Ethnology, Washington, D.C., 1946, 486.

15. Mori, N.; Sakanoue, M.; Takeuchi, M.; Shimpo, K.; and Tanabe, T., *Shokuhin Eiseigaku Zassi* 22, 1981, 409.

16. Oliveira Filho, R. M., et al., *General Pharmacology,* Vol. 20, 1989, 187.

17. Yodyingyuad, V., and Bunyawong, S., *Effect of Stevioside on Growth and Reproduction,* Oxford University Press, 1991, 158–65.

18. Sahelian and Gates, op. cit., 29–30.

19. Yodyingyuad and Bunyawong, op. cit.

20. Phillips, op. cit., 7.

21. Wingard, R. E., Jr.; Brown, J. P.; Enderlin, F. E.; Dale, J. A.;

Hale, R. L.; and Seitz, C. T., "Intestinal Degradation and Absorption of the Glycosidic Sweeteners Stevioside and Rebaudioside A," *Experientia,* 1980, 36.

22. Kinghorn and Soejarto, op. cit., 1982, 26, 30.

23. Kinghorn, op. cit., 1992, 26.

24. Mowrey, Daniel B., Ph.D., "Life with Stevia: How Sweet It Is!" Marketing Management Systems, Inc. Mesa, AZ, 1992.

25. Phillips, op. cit., 12.

26. Pezzuto, John M.; Compadre, Cesar; Swanson, Steven M.; Dhammika Nanayakkara, N.P.; and Kinghorn, A. D., "Metabolically Activated Steviol, the Aglycone of Stevioside, Is Mutagenic," *Medical Science,* 1983.

27. Ibid.

28. Ibid.

29. Shubik, Philippe, *Toxicological Review of Stevia Rebaudiana,* Green College, University of Oxford, 9–10.

30. Pezzuto et al., op. cit.

31. Toyoda, K.; Matsui, H.; Shoda, T.; Uneyama, C.; Takada, K.; and Takahashi, M., *Assessment of the Carcinogenicity of Stevioside in F344 Rats,* Elsevier Science Ltd., London, 1997, 597–603.

32. Sahelian and Gates, op. cit. 30–31.

CHAPTER 8

1. Scientific Committee on Food, Opinion on *Stevia Rebaudiana Bertoni* Plants and Leaves, June 17, 1999.

2. Ibid.

3. Scientific Committee on Food, Opinion on Stevioside as a Sweetener, June 17, 1999.

4. Ibid.

CHAPTER 9

1. Monte, Woodrow C., Ph.D., R.D., "Aspartame: Methanol and the Public Health," *Journal of Applied Nutrition,* Vol. 36, 42, 1984.

2. Whitaker, Julian, M.D., "The Lowdown on Aspartame (Nutra-Sweet)," *Health and Healing,* Vol. 12, No. 3, March 2000, 1–3.

3. Roberts, H. J., M.D., *Aspartame (NutraSweet): Is It Safe?*, The Charles Press, Philadelphia, 1990, 26–28.

4. Ibid., 32–33.

5. Ibid., 31.

6. Ibid., 35.

7. Ibid., 35–36.

8. Ibid., 36.

9. Monte, op. cit., 44.

10. Roberts, op. cit., 37–39.

11. Monte, op. cit., 46.

12. Ibid., 44.

13. Idid., 44–45.

14. Whitaker, op. cit., 2.

15. Ibid.

16. Ibid.

CHAPTER 10

1. *FDA Consumer*, October 1988, 17.

2. *FDA Consumer*, September 1981.

3. Monte, op. cit., 42.

4. Strubbe, Bill, "Killing Me Sweetly . . . How Safe Is Aspartame?," www.salon.com.

5. *Federal Register,* July 24, 1981, 38289.

6. *Congressional Record-Senate,* May 7, 1985, S5493.

7. Roberts, op. cit., 2.

8. Strubbe, op. cit.

9. Ibid.

10. Ibid.

11. Ibid.

12. Ibid.

13. *FDA* Consumer, *Food Allergies Rare but Risky*, May 1994.

14. *FDA* Consumer, "Sugar Substitutes: Americans Opt for Sweetness and Lite," November–December 1999.

15. Strubbe, op. cit.

16. Monte, op. cit.

17. Monte, op. cit., 42.

18. Roberts, op. cit, 46.

19. Ibid., 47.

20. Ibid., 87–89.

21. Strubbe, op. cit., 4–5.

22. Roberts, op. cit., 89.

23. Ibid., 236.

24. Roberts, op. cit., 236.

25. Ibid.

26. Roberts, op. cit., 255, 241.

27. Ibid.

28. Ibid., 242.

29. Roberts, H. J., *Aspartame Disease: An Ignored Epidemic,* Sunshine Sentinel Press, West Palm Beach, FL, 2001.

30. Whitaker, "The lowdown on Aspartame (Nutrasweet)," op. cit., 1–3.

Chapter 12

1. Grigg, William, *FDA Consumer,* November 1988, 30.

2. Ibid., 30.

3. Ibid., 32.

4. Ibid., 31–32.

5. Grigg, William, *FDA Consumer,* December 1988/January 1989, 28.

6. Ibid., 28–30.

7. The account of this event was gleaned from personal conversations with Dr. Wright, members of his staff, eyewitnesses, and a series of articles published in *Health Freedom News,* June and July/August 1992.

Chapter 13

1. Bonvie, Linda, and Bill Bonvie, "Sinfully Sweet," *New Age Journal,* January–February 1996, 120.

2. Ibid., 62

3. Ibid.

4. Ibid.

5. Kinghorn, A. D., Ph.D., (Ed.), *Stevia, The Genus Stevia,* Taylor and Francis, London, 2002, 12.

6. FDA Import Alert, No. 45–06, Regulatory Procedure Manual Part 9, Imports, Chapter 9–79, May 17, 1991.

7. Blumenthal, Mark, "Perspectives of FDA's New Stevia Policy," *Whole Foods Magazine,* February 1996, 70.

8. Ibid.

9. Bonvie, op cit.

10. Mowrey, op cit.

CONCLUSION

1. Folz, C. F., *Bolivia Stevia Development Project: A Commercial Viability Study,* September 1996, 21.

INDEX